A PRACTICAL GUIDE
TO
INTEGRAL YOGA

(*Extracts compiled from the writings of Sri Aurobindo and The Mother*)

SRI AUROBINDO ASHRAM
PONDICHERRY

First Edition: 1955
Reprinted: 1958, 1959, 1965, 1971, 1973

Seventh Edition (Facsimile): 1976
Reprinted: 1985, 1991, 1995, 1998

ISBN 81-7058-034-X

Pub

LOTUS LIGHT
PUBLICATIONS
Box 325
Twin Lakes, WI 53181 USA

THIS WORK
I DEDICATE AT THE LOTUS FEET
OF THE DIVINE MOTHER,
THE SOLE MASTER OF MY BEING

One who truly follows the path laid out by Sri Aurobindo, as soon as he begins to have the experience of this path, would find it impossible to reduce his consciousness to the cult of any god or goddess whatever.

⁂

Those who still believe in gods can certainly continue to worship them if they feel like it — but they must know that this creed and this worship has nothing to do with the teaching of Sri Aurobindo and no connection whatever with the Supramental Realisation.

⁂

I do not see any necessity for us to worship gods, big or small. Our adoration must go only to the Supreme Lord.

⁂

Sri Aurobindo is a permanent Avatar of the Lord.

The Mother

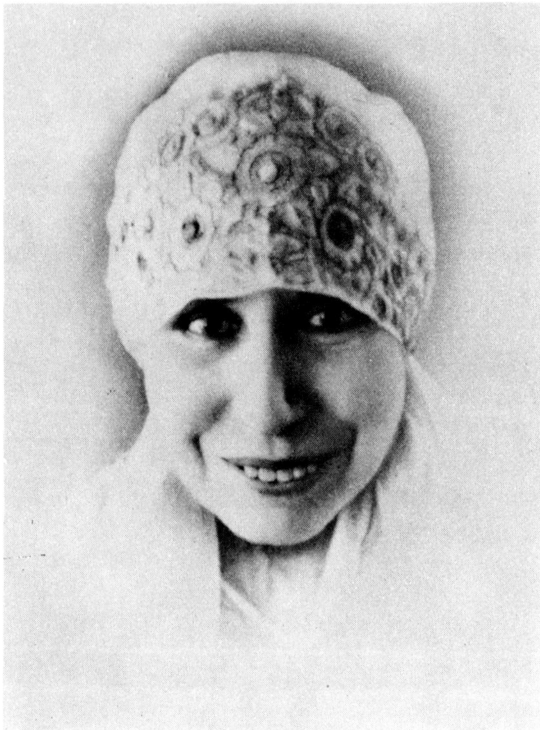

THE DIVINE MOTHER

Born : 21-2-1878 *Withdrawn : 17-11-1973*

Lord, Thou hast willed, and I execute:
A new light breaks upon the earth,
A new world is born.
The things that were promised are fulfilled.

The Mother

The Mother's consciousness and mine are the same, the one Divine Consciousness in two, because that is necessary for the play. Nothing can be done without her knowledge and force, without her consciousness.

Sri Aurobindo

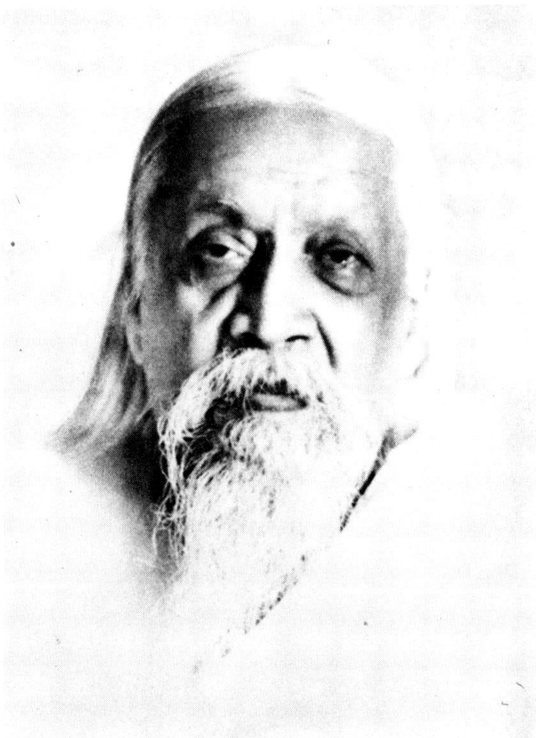

SRI AUROBINDO

The Divine Master

Born : 15-8-1872 *Withdrawn : 5-12-1950*

The one and the only aim we have before us is to bring down the supramental Consciousness and the supramental Truth into the world; the truth and nothing but the Truth is our aim, and if we cannot embody this Truth, a hundred incarnations do not matter.

*

By this Yoga we not only seek the Infinite, but we call upon the Infinite to unfold himself in human life.

Sri Aurobindo

CONTENTS

Section One

Section Two

Section Three

APPENDIX

SECTION ONE

PREFACE

To start with, it is important to know what we as human beings are and what our life is.

Under the Divine Wisdom, the earth has evolved from matter to plant life and then to animal life. Evolution from animal to man is not the final stage. Humanity is under the sway of dark and ignorant forces and that is the reason for human sufferings, disease and death — all the signs of imperfection. It is clear that man has to progress towards a Light which brings knowledge, power, happiness, love, beauty and even physical immortality. The Divine is the essence of the whole universe and to realise and possess Him should be the supreme aim of human life. To acquire all the qualities of the Divine is the final purpose of Nature's evolution.

Mere ideas and ideals, mere talk about God and the Good cannot help. Nor can performance of religious rites really help. A firm resolution should spring from one's heart to realise the Divine, and nothing else should matter. Emotional enthusiasm does not by itself go very far. One must be ready to pass through the hard ordeals of the spiritual path. One cannot persist to the end unless one keeps the will firm and draws on the support of an inner strength.

The soul progresses by gathering experiences in the ordinary life but it is a very long, slow and devious process from birth to birth. Yoga hastens the soul's development. The progress that can be made in many lives is made in a few years by the help of Yoga.

Just as modern science has advanced greatly over past researches and brought new truths and powers, the Yoga of Sri Aurobindo and the Mother has also made a momentous advancement over all past Yogas. It is called the "Integral Yoga" or the "Supramental Yoga".

Where the past Yogas end, this new Integral Yoga starts. The Yogas of the past were only of ascent to the Spirit, Sri Aurobindo's Yoga is both of ascent and descent. One can realise the Divine in consciousness by the old Yogas but cannot establish the Divine on earth in a collective no less than in an individual physical life. In the old Yogas the world was considered either an illusion or a tran-

sitional phase : it had no prospect of having all the terms of its existence fulfilled. Sri Aurobindo says that the world is a real creation of the Divine and life in it can be completely divinised, down to the very cells of the body. A Kingdom of God on earth can be brought about in the most literal sense by a total transformation of collective men.

To put it in Sri Aurobindo's words : "Here and not elsewhere the highest Godhead has to be found, the soul's divine nature developed out of the imperfect physical human nature and through unity with God and man and universe the whole large truth of being discovered and lived and made visibly wonderful. That completes the long cycle of our becoming and admits us to a supreme result; that is the opportunity given to the soul by the human birth and, until that is accomplished, it cannot cease."

For this transformation a new power called the "Supermind" which was sealed to this earth till now is needed. By its manifestation in earth-nature a supreme evolution is made possible.

The Mother has declared recently that at last the Supermind has manifested. It is now only a question of time to have its increasing effect in world-life. This new Light will work everywhere in general but it will be more effective in those who come into direct contact with the Masters of this Yoga and take up the Yogic life in earnest.

More and more people, in India as well as abroad, are drawn towards Sri Aurobindo and the Mother and are anxious to know their teachings. A need is felt to collect these teachings in a single book which would combine brevity with many-sidedness and serve as an introduction to the new path. We hope the present collection will prove helpful to all sincere aspirants.

MANIBHAI

AN OUTLINE OF INTEGRAL YOGA

We are human beings, the highest kind of creatures in this world, and we think that nothing can be higher than man. Modern Science is the seal of man's capacity. He can even destroy himself and this world, but cannot create a new world. He has developed instruments of immense possibility but only with the development of the consciousness such instruments can be used with advantage. To be free from constant dangers of conflict and destruction the man of today has to grow inwardly as well as outwardly.

In his present condition man lives in ignorance. He does not know how he thinks and how he acts. He has no true goal of life but wastes his whole life driven by passions and endless desires. His life is full of miseries, sufferings, disharmony, discords, disease and death. In fact, man is an animal, a thinking and speaking animal but still an animal in his instincts and habits. The creature of water cannot dream of the creation on land. The animal kingdom though on land cannot get the least idea of man's capacities. So with man also. Man is a creature of this world and he cannot know much of things other than this world. However, he has a capacity in himself to develop to the next stage of evolution because Nature cannot stop with imperfect results and the present humanity must evolve further till the final perfection is obtained. With the final perfection, man's life will be one of knowledge, love, beauty, harmony and joy; quite free from sufferings, miseries, disease and death.

Because we are creatures of this world, our consciousness is always externalised and we look at things and happenings from the outer surface, having no knowledge whatsoever of the real causes and effects of the different forces and influences of the subtle worlds working behind them. We can see and feel only the results on the material plane and nothing more. Our senses have a very limited scope and they can give us the knowledge of the things which are only materialised. But, in fact, that is not all that we are. We have another part in ourselves which is veiled by the external consciousness, and we call that as our Soul — the spark of the Divinity within, which is ONE everywhere — the True Self.

As our senses give us the knowledge of the external things by directing our consciousness outwardly, in the same way if we can direct our consciousness inwardly and rise into the inner consciousness, we can know the things of the higher worlds. We have to take an entire turn in our consciousness and go beyond the limitations of our physical senses, then only can we have the true knowledge of this world and the worlds beyond and that practice is called the 'YOGA'.

All the systems of Yoga practised up to now had almost the same goal and purpose. That is to raise the consciousness to a stage of Bliss and fix it there. They had not much to do with the life here and with this world. They considered this world as an illusion and not worth living in. Yoga was practised for personal salvation and the world at large had no gain out of it. People in the past could not achieve the highest summits of realisation and did not know the purpose of this creation: hence they declared the world to be an illusion.

The Divine, though ONE, has two aspects — one is static and the other dynamic. The dynamic side of the Divine is the energy or the creative side and the Maha Shakti or the Divine Mother stands for it. People in the past realised only the static aspect of the Divine and did not know much of the dynamic side as it is much more difficult to realise it. For this reason, the purpose of the creation was not understood by them and they declared the world to be futile and deceptive. That means either the Divine was unable to make a perfect world and he had no purpose in the creation or man has not been able to understand the same. Sri Aurobindo's Yoga gives the full experience of both the aspects of the Divine, that is why he calls his Yoga the Integral Yoga or the Perfect Yoga. Sri Aurobindo says the Divine is real and His creation is bound to be real. It is only Sri Aurobindo who has shown to the world the purpose of the creation and has declared that the world is still in an imperfect condition and passing through the transitory period towards its perfection. His Yoga teaches one, not only to rise in consciousness but also to bring down the lights and powers of the higher worlds into the lower spheres of consciousness and join both the higher and the lower; then only the Life-Divine can be created and the kingdom of God established on earth.

The meaning of the word 'Yoga', in its true sense is to 'join' — join our external consciousness with our true self — the Divine within ourselves — which is ONE everywhere. By the practice of Yoga, our consciousness expands as wide as the universe and far beyond.

To practise Yoga it is indispensable to have a Guru or a Master, who has a thorough knowledge of the path and a capacity to guide and protect his disciples from all the dangers of the unknown spheres arising either from too powerful lights or from adverse beings of different worlds. The Mother once said : — "Be faithful to your Guru whoever he is, he will lead you as far as you can go. But if you are lucky enough to have the Divine as your Guru then there will be no limit to your realisation".

At a juncture of some new evolution on earth, the Divine takes the lead. He manifests in a form necessary for the purpose and brings a new light with him that will help the evolution and bring about a change in the course of time. Hindus in India believe in such manifestations and also believe that there have been ten manifestations since the beginning of the creation on earth — the first being the Matsya Avatara (the Fish), then Kurma (the Tortoise), then Varaha (the Boar), then Nrisimha (the Man-Lion) and so on. These manifestations show the gradations of evolution on earth. The Fish Manifestation brought a creation in water, the Tortoise brought the first creation on land, the Boar Manifestation brought a creation of developed land animals and the Man-Lion brought a further evolution from animal towards man and so on.

We need, today, a new manifestation which can put the present humanity under a new cosmic power and bring about a new evolution of the present man and the world. Sri Aurobindo once said that the coming evolution will be the final stage for this world. It will be a world of perfect harmony, love, beauty, knowledge and Ananda. The consciousness and the life of the present man will be transformed and a new race will be created.

To effectuate the above result, a new higher power is required to be established upon earth and made native to this world. That power Sri Aurobindo calls the Supramental Power or the Truth-Consciousness. That supramental power alone has the capacity to transform the life of man and change the world conditions. Both the Divine Mother and Sri Aurobindo have manifested upon earth to bring about this new evolution and prepare the necessary conditions on earth for the establishment of the supramental Light. Unless the conditions are created the new Light cannot stay here permanently.

When Divine manifestations take place, they have also to pass through great difficulties and sufferings as a result of oppositions of dark and anti-divine forces which have had a hold upon earth since the creation. Those dark powers always oppose the new Lights because they do not want to give up their grip on the earth and sometimes their hostility even takes the form of war on earth, but in spite of all obstructions the Divine Will succeeds at last. For these reasons, to bring about a radical and collective change, Sri Aurobindo had to take a voluntary decision to leave his body in December 1950, and fight out certain forces in the subtle world. When that conquest on the subtle plane is made and the necessary conditions also are prepared by the Mother in the world atmosphere, Sri Aurobindo, with the help of the Mother, will manifest in a physical form in a divine body without taking a normal human birth. That will be the first supramental body in this world built in the supramental way. Side by side with the first effect of that new Light the Mother's physical body will be transformed and perfected. It will be a fully divinised and immortal body free from disease and death, free from inertia, plastic and luminous with an all-pervading consciousness, perfect knowledge and unlimited powers. The influence of that Divine Manifestation will grow increasingly in the world and change the world conditions and the present earthly life of man. Those who will be ready to receive the new Light will be profited greatly. This is the perfect Yoga for the new evolution which transforms mind, life and body of man.

People in ignorance fall into discussions and say that the Divine is everywhere and ask what the necessity is for the manifestations. In reply it can be said that electricity is everywhere in the atmosphere, as all the scientists declare, and it does work also in the world atmosphere according to the cosmic law; yet, to make the electric power effective for our material use, some conditions are required to be created on the material plane such as dynamos and generators etc. In the same way the Divine also acts in the world atmosphere according to the cosmic law. The Divine is still in a veiled form in this world and has not yet manifested Himself in his full Glory. To establish new Powers and Lights in the world for the evolutionary principles, the Divine has to take a physical form from time to time till the final evolution is effected. Such manifestations serve the purpose of generators and dynamos on the material plane. The Mother herself has said: "Since the beginning of the earth wherever and whenever there was the possibility of manifesting a ray of the Consciousness, I was there". It is the Overmind that governs the earth at present and the higher gods and goddesses belong to that plane of consciousness. Supermind is much higher than Overmind. Sri Aurobindo and the Mother have manifested from the Supramental Plane that is why their powers are much more creative and effective on earth than any god or goddess known to this world.

For the final stage of evolution the Divine will manifest in His full Power in an unveiled form. We may hope that the time is not very far now when Sri Aurobindo will manifest in a divine body with his full Glory, remove all tensions from the world-atmosphere and save the earth.

To begin their Yoga, the first necessities for man are aspiration, faith, devotion, sincerity and rejection of falsehood with a crowning goal of complete and unreserved surrender of the whole being in all its parts — mental, vital and physical, to the Divine alone and to no other influence of the lower Nature.

The more the surrender progresses the more concretely the dynamic and conscious Force of the Divine Mother works for and in the sadhaka and carries out the purification and transformation of the whole being.

As the Divine influence of Sri Aurobindo and the Mother is well established in the whole world atmosphere, the aspirant from any corner of the world can receive the help and protection from them according to the intensity and sincerity of his aspiration and can progress gradually in spirituality.

By sincere aspiration, faith and devotion one can progress in consciousness even at a distance, but for a complete transformation down to the physical it is inevitable to come physically in direct contact of the Masters of this Integral Yoga.

Spirituality is not morality but much higher. Morality is based on human mental standards of good and evil while spirituality is based on the Spirit or the Divine Consciousness. To be one with the Divine Consciousness and Bliss and to act on the physical plane as an outflow of the Divine's Will — to surcharge the whole being with the Supreme and possess all Knowledge, Ananda, Beauty, Power, Love, Harmony and Immortality on the earth itself, — this is the goal of the Integral Yoga.

For a sincere sadhaka it is necessary to be exceedingly careful about his company and environments. You can lose in a few minutes what it has taken you months to gain. Contacts with hostile and undesirable persons and even people of spiritual influence foreign to the Integral Yoga, Holy places, Temples and Churches have an influence adverse to the working of this Yoga and are a hindrance to progress.

MANIBHAI

Sri Aurobindo Ashram
Pondicherry

It matters not if there are hundreds of beings plunged in the densest ignorance. He [Sri Aurobindo] whom we saw yesterday is on earth: His presence is enough to prove that a day will come when darkness shall be transformed into light, when Thy reign shall be indeed established upon earth.

THE MOTHER
30-3-1914

*

Since the beginning of the earth, wherever and whenever there was the possibility of manifesting a ray of the Consciousness, I was there.

THE MOTHER

*

Without him, I exist not;
Without me, he is unmanifest.

THE MOTHER
6-5-1957

*

What Sri Aurobindo represents in the world's history is not a teaching, not even a revelation; it is a decisive action direct from the Supreme.

THE MOTHER

*

LORD, we are upon earth to accomplish Thy work of transformation. It is our sole will, our sole preoccupation. Grant that it may be also our sole occupation and that all our actions may help us towards this single goal.

THE MOTHER

INTRODUCTORY

LIFE'S GOAL

(i)

The ascent to the divine Life is the human journey, the Work of works, the acceptable Sacrifice. This alone is man's real business in the world and the justification of his existence, without which he would be only an insect crawling among other ephemeral insects on a speck of surface mud and water which has managed to form itself amid the appalling immensities of the physical universe.

(ii)

Whoever clings to desires and weaknesses of the flesh, the cravings and passions of the vital in its turbulent ignorance, the dictates of his personal mind unsilenced and unillumined by a greater knowledge, cannot find the true inner law and is heaping obstacles in the way of the divine fulfilment. Whoever is able to detect and renounce those obscuring agencies and to discern and follow the true Guide within and without will discover the spiritual law and reach the goal of the yoga.

(iii)

The Divine Life and the transformation of the lower human into a higher divine nature must be made the sole aim of all the life. No attachment, desire or habit of the mind, heart, vital-being or body should be clung to which come in the way of this one aspiration and one object of life. One must be ready to renounce all these completely as soon as the demand comes from above and the Divine Shakti.

(iv)

First, the consciousness must be transformed, then life, then the forms. It is in this order that the new creation will happen. All Nature's activity is, in fact, a progressive return towards the Supreme Reality which is at once the origin and the goal of the universe, in its totality as well as in its smallest element; we have to become concretely what we are essentially. We must live integrally the truth, the beauty, the power and the perfection hidden in the depth of our being. It is then that all life will become the expression of the sublime, eternal, divine Joy.

(v)

Some give their soul to the Divine, some their life, some offer their work, some their money. A few consecrate all of themselves and all they have — soul, life, work, wealth; these are the true children of God. Others give nothing — these, whatever their position, power and riches, are for the Divine purpose valueless cyphers.

(vi)

The Adverse Powers are the forces and beings that are interested in maintaining the falsehoods they have created in the world of the Ignorance and in putting them forward as the Truth which men must follow. In India they are termed Asuras, Rakshasas, Pishachas who are in opposition to the Gods, the Powers of Light. These too are Powers, for they too have their cosmic field in which they exercise their function and authority and some of them were once divine Powers who have fallen towards the darkness by revolt against the divine Will behind the cosmos.

As for the Mother and myself, we have had to try all the ways, follow all methods, to surmount mountains of difficulties, a far heavier burden to bear than you or anybody else in the Ashram or outside, far more difficult conditions, battles to fight, wounds to endure, ways to cleave through impenetrable morass and desert and forest, hostile masses to conquer — a work such as, I am certain, none else had to do before us. For the leader of the way in a work like ours has not only to bring down or represent and embody the Divine, but to represent too the ascending element in humanity and to bear the burden of humanity to the full and experience, not in a mere play or Lila but in grim earnest, all the obstruction, difficulty, opposition, baffled, hampered and only slowly victorious labour which are possible on the path.... It is because we have the complete experience that we can show a straighter and easier road to others — if they will only consent to take it. It is because of our experience won at a tremendous price that we can urge it upon you and others.

THE LAST DECISIVE BATTLE

(Between the Asuric and the Divine Forces in 1955)

I foresee that the coming year will be a difficult year. There will be much inner struggle and much outer struggle too. So I shall tell you of the attitude you should take in such circumstances.

Indeed the more things become difficult, the quieter you should remain, the more unshakable the faith you should have.

When difficulties come, human beings usually get agitated, excited, nervous and so make the difficulties hundredfold more difficult.

The difficulties may last perhaps more than the twelve months of the year, may extend to fourteen months. It is in the nature of things. The nature of the struggle determines the measure of its duration. The forces must come up to a certain pitch of activity to produce a certain result.

We make use of time in the measure of our small human duration. But naturally Divine Forces have not the same measure as we have and that may appear to us too long or too uncertain. For the Divine, however, that is the shortest way, in spite of everything, to the goal aimed at. The goal is the fulfilment of the Divine Will, whatever it is. Given the circumstances, the Divine always takes the shortest way, although that may seem to us the longest, or tortuous and uncertain. Because we do not see the whole, we see just a little fragment which is according to our proportions. Our vision is narrow, narrow with regard to what is behind, narrow with regard to what is ahead. Man's vision is limited; he cannot see very much beyond his nose. Human vision is linear, that is to say, things present themselves to it one after another in a line. Divine vision is different; it is total, it is global: it looks at the problem integrally, that is to say, from all sides, in the round, not from one side or at one point; the supreme vision takes in all sides and aspects at a glance, not only on the surface, but in the depth too. It embraces all the elements of the question and resolves the question without neglecting any of the points involved in it. Man, on the contrary, follows a straight line; anything that is not on the straight line escapes his notice, and if it were left to his choice, these other things would not get done. The Divine's way is circular and yet it is the most direct.

The adverse forces have always tried to push back the divine Realisation as much as possible, to maintain their hold upon the world as long as possible. That struggle seems now to have come to a head at last. It is their final chance. These forces are not blind or ignorant forces merely, there are conscious beings behind them and they know that it is their last chance; therefore they are putting forth all their will and strength as much as they can and what they can is very great. They are not at all like human beings with their small consciousness and smaller power to which they appear formidable and even as divine forces, not only in the measure of their power, but in their consciousness too. They are engaged in a tremendous battle upon this earth; for it is upon this earth that the victory has to be won, the victory that will decide the course of earth's future.

Those whose heart leaps up, who hold their head high just when things become specially dangerous, will have their full satisfaction. It is now the occasion to surmount oneself.

31-12-1954 THE MOTHER

THE VICTORY

The Lord has willed and Thou dost execute:
A new light shall break upon the earth,
A new world shall be born,
And the things that were promised shall be fulfilled.

25th September, 1914 THE MOTHER

*

Lord, Thou hast willed, and I execute:
A new light breaks upon the earth,
A new world is born.
The things that were promised are fulfilled.

29th February, 1956 THE MOTHER

*

The manifestation of the Supramental upon earth is no more a promise but a living fact, a reality.

It is at work here, and one day will come when the most blind, the most unconscious, even the most unwilling shall be obliged to recognise it.

24th April, 1956 THE MOTHER

*

Open yourself to the new Light that has dawned upon earth and a luminous path will spread in front of you.

28th May, 1956 THE MOTHER

THREE CONCEPTIONS OF THE WORLD

1. BUDDHIST AND SHANKARA:

The world is an illusion, a field of ignorance and suffering due to ignorance. The one thing to do is to get out of it as soon as possible and to disappear into the original Non-Existence or Non-Manifestation.

2. THE VEDANTIC AS VERY COMMONLY UNDERSTOOD:

The world is essentially divine, for the divine is omnipresent there. But its exterior expression is distorted, obscure, ignorant, perverted. The one thing to do is to become conscious of the inner divine and remain fixed in that consciousness without troubling about the world; for this external world cannot change and will always be in its natural state of unconsciousness and ignorance.

3. SRI AUROBINDO'S VIEW:

The world, as it is, is not the divine creation it is meant to be, but an obscure and perverted expression of it. It is not the expression of the divine consciousness and will, but this is what it is meant to become; it has been created to develop into a perfect manifestation of the Divine under all His forms and aspects — Light and Knowledge, Power, Love and Beauty.

This is our conception of it and the aim we follow.

24-2-1936 THE MOTHER

TO THE CHILDREN OF THE ASHRAM

There is an ascending evolution in nature which goes from the stone to the plant, from the plant to the animal, from the animal to man. Because man is, for the moment, the last rung at the summit of the ascending evolution, he considers himself as the final stage in this ascension and believes there can be nothing on earth superior to him. In that he is mistaken. In his physical nature he is yet almost wholly an animal, a thinking and speaking animal, but still an animal in his material habits and instincts. Undoubtedly, nature cannot be satisfied with such an imperfect result; she endeavours to bring out a being who will be to man what man is to the animal, a being who will remain a man in its external form, and yet whose consciousness will rise far above the mental and its slavery to ignorance.

Sri Aurobindo came upon earth to teach this truth to men. He told them that man is only a transitional being living in a mental consciousness, but with the possibility of acquiring a new consciousness, the Truth-consciousness, and capable of living a life perfectly harmonious, good and beautiful, happy and fully conscious. During the whole of his life upon earth, Sri Aurobindo gave all his time to establish in himself this consciousness he called supramental, and to help those gathered around him to realise it.

You have the immense privilege of having come quite young to the Ashram, that is to say, still plastic and capable of being moulded according to this new ideal and thus becoming the representatives of the new race. Here, in the Ashram, you are in the most favourable conditions with regard to the environment, the influence, the teaching and the example, to awaken in yourselves this supramental consciousness and to grow according to its law.

Now, all depends on your will and your sincerity. If you have the will no more to belong to ordinary humanity, no more to be merely evolved animals: if your will is to become men of the new race realising Sri Aurobindo's supramental ideal, living a new and higher life upon a new earth, you will find here all the necessary help to achieve your purpose; you will profit fully by your stay in the Ashram and eventually become living examples for the world.

24-7-1951 THE MOTHER

HUMANITY

Its Present Condition and Need

The whole aim of the material man is to live, to pass from birth to death with as much comfort or enjoyment as may be on the way, but anyhow to live.... The customary routine, the customary institutions, the inherited or habitual forms of thought, — these things are the life-breath of their nostrils.... To the material man the living progressive thinker is an ideologue, dreamer or madman.

*

The surfaces of life are easy to understand; their laws, characteristic movements, practical utilities are ready to our hand and we can seize on them and turn them to account with a sufficient facility and rapidity. But they do not carry us very far. They suffice for an active superficial life from day to day, but they do not solve the great problems of existence.

*

The word civilisation so used comes to have a merely relative significance or hardly any fixed sense at all. We must therefore get rid in it of all that is temporary or accidental and fix it upon this distinction that barbarism is the state of society in which man is almost entirely preoccupied with his life and body, his economic and physical existence.... It is obvious that in a state of barbarism the rude beginnings of civilisation may exist; it is obvious too that in a civilised society a great mass of barbarism or numerous relics of it may exist. In that sense all societies are semi-civilised.

*

Man is an abnormal who has not found his own normality, — he may imagine he has, he may appear to be normal in his own kind, but that normality is only a sort of provisional order; therefore, though man is infinitely greater than the plant or the animal, he is not perfect in his own nature like the plant and the animal. This imperfection is not a thing to be at all deplored, but rather a priviledge and a promise, for it opens out to us an immense vista of self-development and self-exceeding.

*

The Divine is infinite and immortal being; the human is life limited in time and scope and form, life that is death attempting to become life that is immortality.

*

In subhuman life of animal there is a vital and physical struggle, but no mental conflict. Man is subject to this mental conflict and is therefore at war not only with others but with himself; and because he is capable of this war with himself, he is also capable of that which is denied to the animal, of an inner evolution, a progression from higher to higher type, a constant self-transcending.

*

The true business of man upon earth is to express in the type of humanity a growing image of the Divine; whether knowingly or unknowingly, it is to this end that Nature is working in him under the thick veil of her inner and outer processes. But the material or animal man is ignorant of the inner aim of life; he knows only its needs and its desires and he has necessarily no other guide to what is required of him than his own perception of need and his own stirrings and pointings of desire.

*

The Self of man is a thing hidden and occult; it is not his body, it is not his life, it is not — even though he is in the scale of evolution the mental being, the Manu, — his mind. Therefore neither the fullness of his physical, nor of his vital, nor of his mental nature can be either the last term or the true standard of his self-realisation.

*

We miss the divine reality in man and the secret of the human birth if we do not see that each individual man is that Self and sums up all human potentiality in his own being. That potentiality he has to find, develop, work out from within.

*

The knowledge of God is not to be gained by weighing the feeble arguments of reason for or against his existence; it is to be gained only by a self-transcending and absolute consecration, aspiration and experience. Nor does that experience proceed by anything like rational scientific experiment or rational philosophic thinking.

*

Man's road to spiritual supermanhood will be open when he declares boldly that all he has yet developed, including the intellect of which he is so rightly and yet so vainly proud, are now no longer sufficient for him, and that to uncase, discover, set free this greater Light within shall be henceforward his pervading preoccupation.

DIVINE LILA (PLAY)

We play at being bound, we are not really bound. We can be free when God wills; for He, our Supreme Self, is the master of the game, and without His Grace and permission no soul can leave the game.

The command is now. God always keeps for himself a chosen country in which the higher knowledge is through all chances and dangers, by the few or the many, continually preserved, and for the present, in this *caturyuga* at least, that country is India. Whenever He chooses to take the full pleasure of ignorance, of the dualities, of strife and wrath and tears and weakness and selfishness, the tamasic and rajasic pleasures, of the play of the Kali in short, He dims the knowledge in India and puts her down into weakness and degradation so that she may retire into herself and not interfere with this movement of His *līlā*. When he wants to rise up from the mud and *Nārāyaṇa* in man to become once again mighty and wise and blissful, then He once more pours out the knowledge on India and raises her up so that she may give the knowledge with its necessary consequences of might, wisdom and bliss to the whole world. When there is the contracted movement of knowledge, the Yogins in India withdraw from the world and practise Yoga for their own liberation and delight or for the liberation of a few disciples; but when the movement of knowledge again expands and the soul of India expands with it, they come forth once more and work in the world and for the world. Yogins like Janaka, Ajatshatru and Kartavirya once more sit on the thrones of the world and govern the nations.

God's lila in man moves always in a circle, from Satyayuga to Kaliyuga and through Kaliyuga to the Satyayuga, from the age of gold to the age of iron and back again through the iron to the gold.... But the Kaliyuga is not merely evil; in it the necessary conditions are progressively built up for a new Satyayuga, another harmony, a more advanced perfection.

It is only India that can discover the harmony, because it is only by a change — not a mere readjustment — of man's present nature that it can be developed, and such a change is not possible except by Yoga. The nature of man and of things is at present a discord, a harmony that has gone out of tune. The whole heart and action and mind of man must be changed, but from within, not from without, not by political and social institutions, not even by creeds and philosophies, but by realisation of God in ourselves and the world and a remoulding of life by that realisation. This can only be effected by Purna-Yoga, a Yoga devoted to the fulfilment of the divine humanity in ourselves and others.

For this Purna-Yoga, the surrender must be complete. Nothing must be reserved, no desire, no demand, no opinion, no idea that this must be, that cannot be, that this should be and that should not be; — all must be given.

To those who demand from Him, God gives what they demand, but to those who give themselves and demand nothing, He gives everything that they might otherwise have asked or needed and in addition He gives Himself and the spontaneous boons of His love.

You must put aside what you want and wish to know what God wants; distrust what your heart, your passions or your habitual opinions prefer to hold as right and necessary.... The power that governs the world is at least as wise as you and it is not absolutely necessary that you should be consulted or indulged in its management; God is seeing to it.

An almighty love and wisdom are at work for your uplifting. Therefore never be troubled by the time that is being taken, even if it seems very long, but when imperfections and obstructions arise, be *apramatta*, *dhīra*, have the *utsāha*, and leave God to do the rest. Time is necessary. It is a tremendous work that is being done in you, the alteration of your whole human nature into a divine nature, the crowding of centuries of evolution into a few years. You ought not to grudge the time.

The goal marked out for us and the call upon us is to grow into the image of God, to dwell in Him and with Him and be a channel of His joy and might and an instrument of His works. Purified from all that is *aśubha*, transfigured in soul by His touch we have to act in the world as dynamos of that divine electricity and send it thrilling and radiating through mankind, so that wherever one of us stands, hundreds around may become full of His light and force, full of God and full of *ānanda.*

Churches, orders, theologies, philosophies have failed to save mankind because they have busied themselves with intellectual creeds, dogmas, rights and institutions, with *ācāra*, *śuddhi* and *darśana*, as if these could save mankind, and have neglected the one thing needful, the power and purification of the soul.

The reason for which the Avatars descend is to raise up man again and again, developing in him a higher and ever higher humanity, a greater and yet greater development of divine being, bringing more and more of heaven again and again upon the earth until our toil is done, our work accomplished and Sachchidananda fulfilled in all even here, even in this material universe.

AIM AND OBJECT OF OUR YOGA

The aim of our Yoga is to open the consciousness to the Divine and to live in the inner consciousness more and more while acting from it on the external life, to bring the inmost psychic into the front and by the power of the psychic to purify and change the being so that it may become ready for transformation and in union with the Divine Knowledge, Will and Love. Secondly, to develop the Yogic consciousness, i.e., to universalise the being in all the planes, become aware of the cosmic being and cosmic forces and be in union with the Divine on all the planes up to the Overmind. Thirdly, to come into contact with the transcendent Divine beyond the Overmind through the supramental consciousness, supramentalise the consciousness and the nature and make oneself an instrument for the realisation of the dynamic Divine Truth and its transforming descent into the earth-nature.

*

The object of our Yoga is to bring down the supramental consciousness on earth, to fix it there, to create a new race with the principle of the supramental consciousness governing the inner and outer individual and collective life.

*

This Yoga does not mean the rejection of the powers of life, but an inner transformation and a change of the spirit in the life and the use of the powers. These powers are now used in an egoistic spirit and for undivine ends; they have to be used in a spirit of surrender to the Divine and for the purpose of the divine Work.

*

The whole principle of this Yoga is to give oneself entirely to the Divine alone and to nobody and nothing else, and to bring down into ourselves by union with the Divine Mother all the transcendent light, power, wideness, peace, purity, truth-consciousness and Ananda of the Supramental Divine.

*

The Divine gives itself to those who give themselves without reserve and in all their parts to the Divine. For them the calm, the light, the power, the bliss, the freedom, the wideness, the heights of knowledge, the seas of Ananda.

*

Man is shut up at present in his surface individual consciousness and knows the world only through his outward mind and senses and by interpreting their contacts with the world. By Yoga there can open in him a consciousness which becomes one with that of the world; he becomes directly aware of a universal Being, universal states, universal Force and Power, universal Mind, Life, Matter and lives in conscious relations with these things. He is then said to have cosmic consciousness.

*

It is the aim of the sadhana that the consciousness should rise out of the body and take its station above, — spreading in wideness everywhere, not limited to the body.

*

To be a Yogi, a Sannyasi, a Tapaswi is not the object here. The object is transformation, and the transformation can only be done by a force infinitely greater than your own; it can only be done by being truly like a child in the hands of the Divine Mother.

*

The object of our Yoga is to enter into and be possessed by the Divine Presence and Consciousness, to love the Divine for the Divine's sake alone, to be tuned in our nature into the nature of the Divine, and in our will and works and life to be the instrument of the Divine. The Divine alone is our object.

*

Spirit is the crown of universal existence; Matter is its basis; Mind is the link between the two. Spirit is that which is eternal; Mind and Matter are its workings. Spirit is that which is concealed and has to be revealed; mind and body are the means by which it seeks to reveal itself. Spirit is the image of the Lord of the Yoga; mind and body are the means He has provided for reproducing that image in phenomenal existence. All Nature is an attempt at a progressive revelation of the concealed Truth, a more and more successful reproduction of the divine image.

But what Nature aims at for the mass in a slow evolution, Yoga effects for the individual by a rapid revolution. It works by a quickening of all her energies, a sublimation of all her faculties....

Nature seeks the divine in her own symbols: Yoga goes beyond Nature to the Lord of Nature, beyond universe to the Transcendent and can return with the transcendent light and power, with the fiat of the Omnipotent.

*

Here the soul lives in a material universe; of that alone it is immediately conscious; the realisation of its potentialities in that are the problem with which it is concerned. But matter means the involution of the conscious delight of existence in self-oblivious force and in a self-dividing, infinitesimally disaggregated form of substance. Therefore the whole principle and effort of a material world must be the evolution of what is involved and the development of what is undeveloped. Here everything is shut up from the first in the violently working inconscient sleep of material force; therefore the whole aim of any material becoming must be the waking of consciousness out of the inconscient; the whole consummation of a material becoming must be the removal of the veil of matter and the luminous revelation of the entirely self-conscient Being to its own imprisoned soul in the becoming. Since Man is such an imprisoned soul, this luminous liberation and coming to self-knowledge must be his highest object and the condition of his perfection.

The gnostic perfection, spiritual in its nature, is to be accomplished here in the body and takes life in the physical world as one of its fields, even though the gnosis opens to us possession of planes and worlds beyond the material universe. The physical body is therefore a basis of action, *pratiṣṭhā*, which cannot be despised, neglected or excluded from the spiritual evolution: a perfection of the body as the outer instrument of a complete divine living on earth will be necessarily a part of the gnostic conversion.

The Mother:

The general aim to be attained is the advent of a progressing universal harmony, and to individualise the states of being that were never till now conscious in man and, by that, to put the earth in connection with one or more of the fountains of universal force that are still sealed to it.

The only way to become a conscious being, to be oneself, is to unite with the divine Self that is in all. For that, we must, by the aid of concentration, isolate ourselves from external influences. When you are one with the Divinity within, you are one with all things in their depths.

Living among others you should always be a divine example, an occasion offered to them to understand and to enter on the path of the life divine. Nothing more. You should not even have the desire to make them progress; for that too would be something arbitrary.

It is an invaluable possession for every living being to have learnt to know himself and to master himself. To know oneself means to know the motives of one's actions and reactions, the why and the how of all that happens in oneself. To master oneself means to do what one has decided to do, to do nothing but that, not to listen to or follow impulses, desires or fancies.

*

The whole world is in a process of progressive transformation; if you take up the discipline of Yoga, you speed up in yourself this process. The work that would require years in the ordinary course, can be done by Yoga in a few days and even in a few hours.

*

Our goal is not to lose oneself in the Divine Consciousness. The goal is to let the Divine Consciousness penetrate into Matter and transform it.

*

Ours is neither a political nor a social but a spiritual goal. What we want is a transformation of the individual consciousness, not a change of regime or government. For reaching that goal we put no confidence in any human means, however powerful, our trust is in the Divine Grace alone.

*

The eternal Veda is the Truth that dwells within the heart of every being; it can express itself spontaneously either in words or as a luminous will.

If one is to prepare for Yoga by the study of books, this preparation would take rather long. But it goes much quicker when one receives directly a teaching which is at one's disposal in all circumstances....

Indeed they who are predestined receive the help of the inner Guide. At the right moment they come across the book they should read or the person who can give them the right indication....

It goes without saying that it is easier for those who are here in India. India maintains her living tradition. An aspirant for Yoga will always find someone who can give him the teaching. Even the most ignorant and the most uncultured possess in them a vague feeling of what is to be done or what can help. But if you transplant yourself to the West, you will see how difficult it is.... Now the situation is somewhat better, there has been some progress, the light has spread a little everywhere....

Note this particularly, you are given a full freedom of choice; if you decide within yourself that you will reach the goal in this life, you will do so — in that case you can succeed even in twelve months....

It is no reason, however, to lose your time on the way; it is no reason why you should follow all the meanderings of the labyrinth and arrive at the goal, decreased by all that you have lost, spent, wasted on the way. But in any case it is a reason why you should never despair whatever the obstacles and difficulties.

When you have something to do, it is better to do it as quickly as possible, that is my opinion. But there are people who like to lose their time. Perhaps they need turning round and round, falling back, going about in circuitous ways before they arrive where they should arrive. Unfortunately it is exactly people who have this habit of loitering, wandering away from the straight line, that most complain of the way being long; they lament, but they themselves are the artisans of their own misery. But to each his choice.

*

What cannot be acquired or conquered during life can certainly not be done after death. The physical life is the true field for progress and realisation.

PAST YOGAS AND THE INTEGRAL YOGA

The way of Yoga followed here has a different purpose from others, — for its aim is not only to rise out of the ordinary ignorant world-consciousness into the divine consciousness, but to bring the supramental power of that divine consciousness down into the ignorance of mind, life and body, to transform them, to manifest the Divine here and create a divine life in Matter. This is an exceedingly difficult aim and difficult Yoga; to many or most it will seem impossible. All the established forces of the ordinary ignorant world-consciousness are opposed to it and deny it and try to prevent it, and the Sadhak will find his own mind, life and body full of the most obstinate impediments to its realisation. If you can accept the ideal whole-heartedly, face all difficulties, leave the past and its ties behind you and are ready to give up everything and risk everything for this divine possibility, then only can you hope to discover by experience the Truth behind it.

*

Asceticism for its own sake is not the ideal of this Yoga, but self-control in the vital and right order in the material are a very important part of it — and even an ascetic discipline is better for our purpose than a loose absence of true control. Mastery of the material implies in it the right and careful utilisation of things and also a self-control in their use.

Forceful suppression (fasting also comes under the head) stands on the same level as free indulgence; in both cases, the desire remains : in the one it is fed by indulgence, in the other it lies latent and exasperated by suppression.

*

Those who seek the Self by the old Yogas separate themselves from mind, life and body and realise the Self and then they proceed from realisation of Self to Nirvana or some Heaven and abandon life. The Supramental Yoga is necessary for the transformation of terrestrial life and being, not for reaching the Self. One must realise the Self first, only afterwards can one realise the Supermind. This Yoga is "new" because it aims at the integrality of the Divine in this world.

The Sadhak of integral Yoga who stops short at the Impersonal is no longer a sadhak of integral Yoga. Without the action of the integral Divine there is no change of the whole nature. If it were not so, the Mother would not be here and I would not be here if a realisation of the Impersonal were sufficient.... It is only the Supramental that is all-knowledge. All below that from Overmind to Matter is Ignorance.

*

Each man who enters the realms of Yogic experience is free to follow his own way; but this Yoga is not a path for anyone to follow, but only for those who accept to seek the aim, pursue the way pointed out upon which a sure guidance is indispensable. It is idle for anyone to expect that he can follow this road far, — much less go to the end by his own inner strength and knowledge without the true aid or influence. Even the ordinary long-practised Yogas are hard to follow without the aid of the Guru; in this which as it advances goes through untrodden countries and unknown entangled regions, it is quite impossible. As for the work to be done, it also is not a work for any sadhak of any path; it is not, either, the work of the "Impersonal" Divine — who, for that matter, is not an active Power but supports impartially all work in the universe. It is a training ground for those who have to pass through the difficult and complex way of this Yoga and none other. All work here must be done in a spirit of acceptance, discipline and surrender, not with personal demands and conditions, but with a vigilant conscious submission to control and guidance....

The fundamental difference is in the teaching that there is a dynamic divine Truth and that into the present world of Ignorance that Truth can descend, create a new Truth-consciousness and divinise Life. The old Yogas go straight from mind to the absolute Divine, regard all dynamic existence as Ignorance, Illusion or Lila; when you enter the static and immutable Divine Truth, they say, you pass out of cosmic existence....

My aim is to realise and also to manifest the Divine in the world, bringing down for the purpose a yet unmanifested Power, — such as the Supermind.

I have to bring it into the cosmic formula and, if so, I must realise the cosmic Divine and become conscious of the cosmic self and the cosmic forces. But I have to embody it here, — otherwise it is left as an influence only and not a thing fixed in the physical world, and it is through the Divine in the individual alone that this can be done.

*

The aim of this Yoga is an opening to a higher Divine Truth beyond life, mind and body and the transformation of these three things into its image. But that transformation cannot take place, and the Truth itself cannot be known in its own unmistakable spirit, perfect light and real body until the whole of the adhar has been fundamentally and patiently purified, and made plastic and capable of receiving what is beyond the construction of the mind, the desires of the vital being and the habits of the physical consciousness and physical being.

*

It is no part of my Yoga to have nothing to do with the world or with life or to kill the senses or entirely inhibit their action. It is the object of my Yoga to transform life by bringing down into it the Light, Power and Bliss of the Divine Truth and its dynamic certitude. This Yoga is not a Yoga of world-shunning asceticism, but of divine life.

This Yoga accepts the value of cosmic existence and holds it to be a reality; its object is to enter into a higher Truth-Consciousness in which action and creation are the expression not of ignorance and imperfection, but of the Truth, the Light, the Divine Ananda. But for that, surrender of the mortal mind, life and body to that Higher Consciousness is indispensable, since it is too difficult for the mortal human being to pass by its own effort beyond mind to a Supramental Consciousness in which the dynamism is no longer mental but of quite another power. Only those who can accept the call to such a change should enter into this Yoga.

My Yoga is new as compared with the old Yogas:—

(1) Because it aims not at a departure out of world and life into Heaven or Nirvana, but at a change of life and existence, not as something subordinate or incidental, but as a distinct and central object. If there is a descent in other Yogas, yet it is only an incident on the way or resulting from the ascent — the ascent is the real thing. Here the ascent is the first step, but it is a means for the descent. It is the descent of the new consciousness attained by the ascent that is the stamp and seal of the sadhana. Even the Tantra and Vaishnavism end in the release from life; here the object is the divine fulfilment of life.

(2) Because the object sought after is not an individual achievement of the divine realisation for the sake of the individual, but

something to be gained for the earth-consciousness here, a cosmic, not solely a supra-cosmic achievement. The thing to be gained also is the bringing in of a Power of Consciousness (the Supramental) not yet organised or active directly in earth-nature, even in the spiritual life, but yet to be organised and made directly active.

(3) Because a method has been preconised for achieving this purpose which is as total and integral as the aim set before it, viz., the total and integral change of the consciousness and nature, taking up old methods but only as a part action and present aid to others that are distinctive. I have not found this method (as a whole) or anything like it professed or realised in the old Yogas. If I had, I should not have wasted my time in hewing out paths and in thirty years of search and inner creation when I could have hastened home safely to my goal in an easy canter over paths already blazed out, laid down, perfectly mapped, macadamised, made secure and public. Our Yoga is not a retreading of old walks, but a spiritual adventure.

*

The purely monistic Vedantist says, all is Brahman, life is a dream, an unreality, only Brahman exists. One has Nirvana or Mukti, then one lives only till the body falls — after that there is no such thing as life.

What has to be overcome is the opposition of the Ignorance that does not want the transformation of the nature. If that can be overcome, then old spiritual ideas will not form an obstacle.

It is not intended to supramentalise humanity at large, but to establish the principle of the Supramental consciousness in the earth-evolution. If that is done, all that is needed will be evolved by the Supramental Power itself. It is not therefore important that the mission should be wide-spread. What is important is that the thing should be done at all in however small a number; that is the only difficulty.

*

It is in the waking state that this realisation must come and endure in order to be a reality of the life. If experienced in trance it will be a superconscient state only for some part of the inner being but not real to the whole consciousness. Experience and trance have their utility for opening the being and preparing it but it is only when the realisation is constant in the waking state that it is truly possessed. Therefore in this Yoga much value is given to the waking realisation and experience.

*

This is not a Yoga of Bhakti alone; it is or at least it claims to be an integral Yoga, that is, a turning of all the being in all its parts to the Divine, so that the nature also may become one with the nature of the Divine.

*

The object of the sadhana is opening of the consciousness to the Divine and the change of the nature. Meditation or contemplation is one means to this but only one means; bhakti is another; work is another. Chittashuddhi was preached by the Yogins as a first means towards realisation and they got by it the saintliness of the saint and the quietude of the sage but the transformation of the nature of which we speak is something more than that, and this transformation does not come by contemplation alone; works are necessary, Yoga in action is indispensable.

The purpose of the old Yogas is to get away from life to the Divine — so obviously, let us drop Karma. The purpose of this new Yoga is to reach the Divine and bring the fullness of what is gained into life — for that, Yoga by works is indispensable.

*

Veda and Vedanta are one side of the One Truth; Tantra with its emphasis on Shakti is another; in this Yoga all sides of the

Truth are taken up, not in the systematic forms given them formerly but in their essence, and carried to the fullest and highest significance. The integral Yoga needs to develop its own forms and processes, but the ascent of the consciousness through the centres and other Tantric knowledge are there behind the process of transformation to which so much importance is given by me — also the truth that nothing can be done except through the force of the Mother.

*

In our Yoga the Nirvana is the beginning of the higher Truth, as it is the passage from the Ignorance to the higher Truth. The Ignorance has to be extinguished in order that the Truth may manifest.

The Jain philosophy is concerned with individual perfection. Our effort is quite different. We want to bring down the Supermind as a new faculty. Just as the mind is now a permanent state of consciousness in humanity, so also we want to create a race in which the Supermind will be a permanent state of consciousness.

*

The old Yoga demanded a complete renunciation extending to the giving up of the worldly life itself. This Yoga aims instead at a new and transformed life. But it insists as inexorably on a complete throwing away of desire and attachment in the mind, life and body. Its aim is to refound life in the truth of the spirit and for that purpose to transfer the roots of all we are and do from the mind, life and body to a greater consciousness above the mind. All must be given up to the Supreme Master of the Yoga.

The power that works in this Yoga is of a thoroughgoing character and tolerates in the end nothing great or small, that is an obstacle to the Truth and its realisation.

*

The traditions of the past are very great in their own place, in the past, but I do not see why we should merely repeat them and not go farther. In the spiritual development of the consciousness upon earth the great past ought to be followed by a greater future.

*

All other Yogas regard this life as an illusion or a passing phase; the supramental Yoga alone regards it as a thing created by the Divine for progressive manifestation and takes the fulfilment of the life and the body for its object.

*

I have objected in the past to *vairāgya* of the ascetic kind and the tamasic kind. I object to it for those who come to this Yoga because it is incompatible with my aim which is to bring the Divine into life.

*

By Yoga we can rise out of falsehood into truth, out of weakness into force, out of pain and grief into bliss, out of bondage into freedom, out of death into immortality, out of darkness into light, out of confusion into purity, out of imperfection into perfection, out of self-division into unity, out of Maya into God. All other utilisation of Yoga is for special and fragmentary advantages not always worth pursuing. Only that which aims at possessing the fullness of God is Purna Yoga or Integral Yoga.

All Yoga which takes us entirely away from the world, is a high but narrow specialisation of divine tapasya. God in His perfection embraces everything, we also must become all-embracing.

In brief, by Yoga, we have to replace dualities by unity, egoism by divine consciousness, ignorance by divine wisdom, thought by divine knowledge, weakness, struggle and effort by self-contented divine force, pain and false pleasure by divine bliss. This is called in the language of Christ bringing down the kingdom of heaven on earth, or in modern language, realising and effectuating God in the world.

*

The principle of this Yoga is not a perfection of human nature as it is, but a psychic and spiritual transformation of all the parts of the being through the action of an inner consciousness and then of a higher consciousness which works on them, throws out the old movements or changes them into an image of its own and so transmutes the lower into higher nature. It is not so much the perfection of the intellect as a transformation of it, a transformation of the mind, the substitution of a larger greater principle of knowledge — and so with all the rest of the being.

This is a slow and difficult process; the road is long and it is hard to establish even the necessary basis. The old existing nature resists and obstructs and difficulties rise one after another, till they are overcome.

Yoga of the Gita

Our Yoga is not identical with the Yoga of the Gita although it contains all that is essential in the Gita's Yoga. In our Yoga we begin with the idea, the will, the aspiration of the complete surrender; but at the same time we have to reject the lower nature, deliver our consciousness from it, deliver the self involved in the lower nature by the self rising to freedom in the higher nature. The full truth is in the supramental consciousness and the power to work from there on life and Matter.

The Gita does not speak expressly of the Divine Mother; it speaks always of surrender to the Purushottama — it mentions her only as the Para Prakriti who becomes the Jiva, that is, who manifests the Divine in the multiplicity and through whom all these worlds are created by the Supreme and he himself descends as the Avatar. The Gita follows the Vedantic tradition which leans entirely on the Ishwara aspect of the Divine and speaks little of the Divine Mother because its object is to draw back from world-nature and arrive at the supreme realisation beyond it; the Tantric tradition leans on the Shakti or Ishwari aspect and makes all depend on the Divine Mother because its object is to possess and dominate the world-nature and arrive at the supreme realisation through it. This Yoga insists on both the aspects; the surrender to the Divine Mother is essential for without it there is no fulfilment of the object of the Yoga.

*

The Gita at its cryptic close may seem by its silence to stop short of that solution for which we are seeking; it pauses at the borders of the highest spiritual mind and does not cross them into the splendours of the supramental Light.

*

It is not a fact that the Gita gives the whole base of Sri Aurobindo's message; for the Gita seems to admit the cessation of birth in the world as the ultimate aim or at least the ultimate culmination of Yoga; it does not bring forward the idea of spiritual evolution or the idea of the higher planes and the supramental Truth-Consciousness and the bringing down of that consciousness as the means of the complete transformation of earthly life....

It is these things among others that constitute the novelty of Sri Aurobindo's message as compared with the Hindu tradition — the idea that the world is not either a creation of Maya or only a play, *līlā*, of the Divine, or a cycle of births in the ignorance from which we have to escape, but a field of manifestation in which there is a progressive evolution of the soul and the nature in Matter and from Matter through Life and Mind till it reaches the complete revelation of Sachchidananda in life. It is this that is the basis of this Yoga and gives a new sense to life.

*

I suggested the Gita method for you because the opening which is necessary for the Yoga here seems to be too difficult for you. I may say that the way of the Gita is itself a part of the Yoga here and those who have followed it, to begin with or as a first stage, have a stronger basis than others for this Yoga.

The ordinary life consists in work for personal aim and satisfaction of desire under some mental or moral control, touched sometimes by a mental ideal. The Gita's Yoga consists in the offering of one's work as a sacrifice to the Divine, the conquest of desire, egoless and desireless action, bhakti for the Divine, an entering into the cosmic consciousness, the sense of unity with all creatures, oneness with the Divine. This Yoga adds the bringing down of the supramental Light and Force and the transformation of the nature.

AVATARHOOD (MANIFESTATION)

An Avatar, roughly speaking, is one who is conscious of the presence and power of the Divine born in him or descended into him and governing from within his will and life and action; he feels identified inwardly with this divine power and presence. But a Vibhuti is supposed to embody some power of the Divine and is enabled by it to act with great force in the world, but that is all that is necessary to make him a Vibhuti: the power may be very great, but the consciousness is not that of an inborn or indwelling Divinity.

The Avatar takes upon himself the nature of humanity in his instrumental parts, though the consciousness acting behind is divine. That does not prevent the Avatar from acting as men act and using the movements of Nature for his life and work. Surely for the earth consciousness the very fact that the Divine manifests himself is the greatest of all splendours.

*

The Divine puts on an appearance of humanity, assumes the outward human nature in order to tread the path and show it to human beings, but does not cease to be the Divine. It is a manifestation that takes place, a manifestation of a growing Divine consciousness, not human turning into divine. The Mother was inwardly above the human even in childhood.

*

When the Divine descends, he takes upon himself the burden of humanity in order to exceed it — he becomes human in order to show humanity how to become Divine. But that cannot be if there is only a weakling without any divine Presence within or divine Force behind him — he has to be strong in order to put his strength into all who are willing to receive it. There is therefore in him a double element — human in front, Divine behind. The Divinity acts according to another consciousness, the consciousness of the Truth above and the Lila below and It acts according to the need of the Lila, not according to men's ideas of what It should or should not do.

The Divine Manifestation, even when it manifests in mental and human ways, has behind it a consciousness greater than the mind and not bound by the petty mental and moral conventions of this very ignorant human race — so that to impose these standards on the Divine is to try to do what is irrational and impossible.

*

The Divine does the sadhana first for the world and then gives what is brought down to others. Naturally, the Mother does the sadhana in each sadhak — only it is conditioned by their zeal and their receptivity.

*

It is much easier for the sadhak by faith in the Mother to keep free — because the Mother by the very nature of her work had to identify herself with the sadhaks, to support all their difficulties, to receive into herself all the poison in their nature, to take up besides all the difficulties of the universal earth-nature, including the possibility of death and disease in order to fight them out. If she had not done that, not a single sadhak would have been able to practise this Yoga. The Divine has to put on humanity in order that the human being may rise to the Divine. — It is a simple truth, but nobody seems to be able to understand that the Divine can do that and yet remain different from them — can still remain the Divine.

*

The Avatar is not supposed to act in a non-human way — he takes up human action and uses human methods with the human consciousness in front and the Divine behind. If he did not, his taking a human body would have no meaning and would be of no use to anybody. He could just as well have stayed above and done things from there.

*

The manifestation of the Divine in the Avatar is of help to man because it helps him to discover his own divinity, find the way to realise it.

There are two sides of the phenomenon of Avatarhood, the Divine Consciousness and the instrumental personality. The Divine Consciousness is omnipotent but it has put forth the instrumental personality in Nature under the conditions of Nature and it uses it according to the rules of the game — though also sometimes to change the rules of the game.

The Divine does not need to suffer or struggle for himself; if he takes on these things it is in order to bear the world-burden and help the world and men. The Divine bears them and at the same time shows the way out of them; otherwise his assumption of human nature has no meaning and no utility and no value. I have said that the Avatar is one who comes to open the Way for humanity to a higher consciousness.

The Mother:

The Divine Grace alone has the power to intervene and change the course of Universal Justice. The great work of the Avatar is to manifest the Divine Grace upon earth. To be a disciple of the Avatar is to become an instrument of the Divine Grace. The Mother is the great dispensatrix — through identity — of the Divine Grace, with a perfect knowledge — through identity — of the absolute mechanism of Universal Justice.

*

The chief purpose of avatarhood is to give to men a concrete proof that the Divine can live upon earth.

*

To believe or not to believe in the possibility of avatarhood can make no difference to the bare fact. If God chooses to manifest in a human body I do not see how any human thought, approval or disapproval can affect in the least His decision; and if He takes birth in a body, the denial of men cannot prevent the fact from being a fact, and if He decides not to incarnate in a human body, the faith, certitude and belief of all humanity cannot in the least alter the fact that He is not incarnate. It is only in perfect quietness and silence, free from all prejudices and preferences, that the consciousness can perceive the truth.

*

In the eternity of becoming each Avatar is only the announcer, the forerunner of a more perfect future realisation.

And yet men have always the tendency to deify the Avatar of the past in opposition to the Avatar of the future.

SRI AUROBINDO ON HIMSELF

For myself, the dark conditions do not discourage me or convince me of the vanity of my will to "help the world", for I knew they had to come; they were there in the world-nature and had to rise up so that they might be exhausted or expelled and a better world freed from them might be there. After all, something has been done in the outer field and that may help or prepare for getting something done in the inner field also. For instance, India is free and her freedom was necessary if the Divine Work was to be done. The difficulties that surround her now and may increase for a time, especially with regard to the Pakistan imbroglio, were also things that had to come and to be cleared out .... Here too there is sure to be a full clearance, though unfortunately, a considerable amount of human suffering in the process is inevitable. Afterwards the work for the Divine will become more possible and it may well be that the dream, if it is a dream, of leading the world towards the spiritual light, may even become a reality. So I am not disposed even now, in these dark conditions to consider my will to help the world as condemned to failure.

*

I believe the descent of this Truth opening the way to a development of divine consciousness here to be the final sense of the earth evolution. If greater men than myself have not had this vision and this ideal before them, that is no reason why I should not follow my Truth-sense and Truth-vision. There is no question of X or Y or anybody else in that. It is a question between the Divine and myself — whether it is the Divine Will or not, whether I am sent to bring that down or open the way for its descent or at least make it more possible or not.

I have no intention of achieving the Supermind for myself only — I am not doing anything for myself, as I have no personal need of anything, neither of salvation (Moksha) nor supramentalisation. If I am seeking after supramentalisation, it is because it is a thing that has to be done for the earth-consciousness and if it is not done in myself, it cannot be done in others. My supramentalisation is only a key for opening the gates of the Supramental to the earth-consciousness; done for its own sake, it would be perfectly futile....

Of course, anyone who wants to change earth-nature must first accept it in order to change it. To quote from a poem of my own, *A God's Labour:—*

> He who would bring the heavens here,
> Must descend himself into clay
> And the burden of earthly nature bear
> And tread the dolorous way....

*

As for faith, you write as if I never had a doubt or any difficulty. I have had worse than any human mind can think of. It is not because I have ignored difficulties, but because I have seen them more clearly, experienced them on a larger scale than anyone living now or before me that, having faced and measured them, I am sure of the results of my work. In the way that one treads with the greater Light above, even every difficulty gives its help and has its value and Night itself carries in it the burden of the Light that has to be.

I know with absolute certitude that the Supramental is a truth and that its advent is in the very nature of things inevitable. The question is as to the when and the how. That also is decided and predestined from somewhere above; but it is here being fought out amid a rather grim clash of conflicting forces. That is, however, certain that a number of souls have been sent to see that it shall be now. My faith and will are for the now.

*

If we had lived physically in the Supermind from the beginning nobody could have been able to approach us nor could any sadhana have been done. There could have been no hope of contact between ourselves and the earth and men. Even as it is, Mother has to come down towards the lower consciousness of the sadhaks instead of keeping always in her own. The Divine has to veil himself in order to meet the human.

*

There is no difference between the Mother's path and mine; we have and always had the same path, the path that leads to the supramental change and the divine realisation; not only at the end, but from the beginning they have been the same.

The attempt to set up a division and opposition putting the Mother on one side and myself on another and opposite or quite different side, has always been a trick of the forces of Falsehood when they want to prevent a sadhak from reaching the Truth. Dismiss all such falsehoods from your mind. The Mother and myself stand for the same Power in two forms.

You consider that the Mother can be of no help to you. If you cannot profit by her help, you would find still less profit in mine. But, in any case, I have no intention of altering the arrangement I have made for all the disciples without exception that they should receive the light and force from her and not directly from me and be guided by her in their spiritual progress. I have made the arrangement not for any temporary purpose but because it is the one way, provided always the disciple is open and receives.

*

The Mother and myself deal with all according to the law of

the Divine. We receive alike rich and poor, those who are high-born or low-born according to human standards, and extend to them an equal love and protection. Their progress in sadhana is our main concern — for they have come here for that, not to satisfy their palates or their bellies, not to make ordinary vital demands or to quarrel about position or place or comforts. That progress depends on how they answer to the Mother's love or protection — whether they receive the forces she pours on all alike, whether they use or misuse what she gives them. But the Mother has no intention or obligation to deal with all outwardly in the same way — the demand that she should do so is absurd and imbecile — and if she did it, she would prove false to the truth of things and the law of the Divine. Each sadhak has to be dealt with according to his nature, his capacities, his real needs (not his claims or desires) and according to what is best for his spiritual welfare. As to how it is to be done, we refuse to be dictated to by the ignorance of those of the sadhaks who consider that the Mother must act according to their standards or their ideas of equality or justice or the demands of their vital or the notions they have brought with them from the outside world. We act according to the Light within us and for the Truth that we are striving to establish in this earthly Nature.

*

In Mother's childhood visions she saw myself whom she knew as "Krishna".

*

The detail of method of the later stages of the Yoga, which go into little known or untrodden regions, I have not made public and I do not at present intend to do so.

What we are doing, if and when we succeed, will be a beginning, not a completion. It is the foundation of a new consciousness on earth — a consciousness with infinite possibilities of manifestation. The eternal progression is in the manifestation and beyond it there is no progression.

*

It is only Divine Love which can bear the burden I have to bear, that all have to bear who have sacrificed everything else to the one aim of uplifting earth out of its darkness towards the Divine....

The Mother's difficulties are not her own; she bears the difficulties of others and those that are inherent in the general action and working for the transformation....

We have to do it through ourselves first and, through the circle of sadhaks gathered around us, in the terrestrial consciousness as typified here. If a few open, that is sufficient for the process to be possible. On the other hand, if there is a general misunderstanding and resistance, that makes it difficult and the process more laborious, but it does not make it impossible.

Progress might be slow at first, but progress would come; it would quicken afterwards and with the supramental force here, there would be for you as for others the full speed and certitude.

*

We are not working for a race or a people or a continent or for a realisation of which only Indians or only Orientals are capable. Our aim is not, either, to found a religion or a school of philosophy or a school of Yoga, but to create a ground of spiritual growth and experience and a way which will bring down a greater Truth beyond the mind but not inaccessible to the human soul and consciousness. All can pass who are drawn to that Truth, whether they are from India or elsewhere, from the East or from the West.

*

It would be only myself who could speak of things in my past giving them their true form and significance.

Neither you nor anyone else knows anything at all of my life; it has not been on the surface for men to see.

*

I may say also that I did not leave politics because I felt I could do nothing more there; such an idea was very far from me. I came away because I got a distinct "Adesh" in the matter....

For the rest, I have never known any will of mine for one major event in the conduct of the world affairs to fail in the end, although it may take a long time for the world-forces to fulfil it.

*

August 15th is my own birthday and it is naturally gratifying to me that it should have assumed this vast significance [of free India]. I take this coincidence, not as a fortuitous accident, but as the sanction and seal of the Divine Force that guides my steps on the work with which I began life, the beginning of its full fruition.... In all these movements free India may well play a large part and take a leading position....

Indeed, on this day I can watch almost all the world-movements which I hoped to see fulfilled in my lifetime, though then they looked like impracticable dreams, arriving at fruition or on their way to achievement.

The first of these dreams was a revolutionary movement which would create a free and united India. India today is free but she has not achieved unity.... The old communal division into Hindus and Muslims seems now to have hardened into a permanent political division of the country. It is to be hoped that this settled fact will not be accepted as settled for ever or as anything more than a temporary expedient. For if it lasts, India may be seriously weakened, even crippled.... This must not be; the partition must go.... By whatever means, in whatever way, the division must go; unity must and will be achieved, for it is necessary for the greatness of India's future.

Another dream was for the resurgence and liberation of the peoples of Asia and her return to her great role in the progress of human civilisation.

The third dream was a world-union forming the outer basis of a fairer, brighter and nobler life for all mankind. That unification of the human world is under way; there is an imperfect initiation organised but struggling against tremendous difficulties.

Another dream, the spiritual gift of India to the world has already begun. India's spirituality is entering Europe and America in an ever increasing measure....

The final dream was a step in evolution which would raise man to a higher and larger consciousness and begin the solution of the problems which have perplexed and vexed him since he first began to think and to dream of individual perfection and a perfect society.

From Early Letters of 1911-1915:

I am developing the necessary powers for bringing down the spiritual on the material plane, and I am now able to put myself into men and change them, removing the darkness and bringing light, giving them a new heart and a new mind. This I can do with great swiftness and completeness with those who are near me, but I have also succeeded with men hundreds of miles away. I have also been given the power to read men's characters and hearts, even their thoughts, but this power is not yet absolutely complete, nor can I use it always and in all cases. My communication with the other world is yet of a troubled character, though I am certainly in communication with some very great powers. But of all these things I will write more when the final obstacles in my way are cleared from the path.

What I perceive more clearly, is that the principal object of my Yoga is to remove absolutely and entirely every possible source of error and ineffectiveness, of error in order that the Truth I shall eventually show to men may be perfect, and of ineffectiveness in order that the work of changing the world, so far as I have to assist it, may be entirely victorious and irresistible. It is for this reason that I have been going through so long a discipline and that the more brilliant and mighty results of Yoga have been so long withheld. I have been kept busy laying down the foundation, a work severe and painful. It is only now that the edifice is beginning to rise upon the sure and perfect foundation that has been laid.

My Yoga is proceeding with great rapidity, but I defer writing to you of the results until certain experiments in which I am now engaged, have yielded fruit sufficient to establish beyond dispute the theory and system of Yoga which I have formed and which is giving great results not only to me, but to the young men who are with me.... I expect these results within a month, if all goes well.

*

The whole earth is now under one law and answers to the same vibrations and I am sceptical of finding any place where the clash of the struggle will not pursue us. In any case, an effective retirement does not seem to be my destiny. I must remain in touch with the world until I have either mastered adverse circumstances or succumbed or carried on the struggle between the spiritual and physical so far as I am destined to carry it on. This is how I have always seen things and still see them.

One needs to have a calm heart, a settled will, entire self-abnegation and the eyes constantly fixed on the beyond to live undiscouraged in times like these which are truly a period of universal decomposition. For myself, I follow the Voice and look neither to the right nor to the left of me. The result is not mine and hardly at all now even the labour.

*

Heaven we have possessed, but not the earth; but the fullness of the Yoga is to make, in the formula of the Veda, "Heaven and Earth equal and one."

*

Everything internal is ripe or ripening, but there is a sort of locked struggle in which neither side can make a very appreciable advance, the spiritual force insisting against the resistance disputing every inch and making more or less effective counter-attacks.... And if there were not the strength and Ananda within, it would be harassing and disgusting work; but the eye of knowledge looks beyond and sees that it is only a protracted episode.

SRI AUROBINDO ON THE MOTHER

The One whom we adore as the Mother is the divine Conscious Force that dominates all existence, one and yet so many-sided that to follow her movement is impossible even for the quickest mind and for the freest and most vast intelligence. The Mother is the consciousness and force of the Supreme and far above all she creates.

But personally too the Mother has stooped to descend here into the Darkness that she may lead it to the Light, into the Falsehood and Error that she may convert it to the Truth, into this Death that she may turn it to godlike Life, into this world-pain and its obstinate sorrow and suffering that she may end it in the transforming ecstasy of her sublime Ananda. In her deep and great love for her children she has consented to put on herself the cloak of this obscurity, condescended to bear the attacks and torturing influences of the powers of the Darkness and the Falsehood, borne to pass through the portals of the birth that is a death, taken upon herself the pangs and sorrows and sufferings of the creation, since it seemed that thus alone could it be lifted to the Light and Joy and Truth and eternal Life.

*

The Mother's consciousness and mine are the same, the one Divine Consciousness in two, because that is necessary for the play. Nothing can be done without her knowledge and force, without her consciousness — if anybody really feels her consciousness, he should know that I am there behind it and if he feels me it is the same with hers.

The Mother's consciousness is the divine consciousness and the Light that comes from it is the light of the Divine Truth. One who receives and accepts and lives in the Mother's light, will begin to see the truth on all the planes, the mental, the vital, the physical.

*

It is not necessary for us always to be physically conscious of the action, for it is often carried out when the mind is occupied with outward things or when we sleep. The Mother's sleep is not sleep but an inner consciousness in which she is in connection with people or working everywhere. At the time she is aware, but she does not carry all that always into her waking consciousness or in her memory. A call would come in the occupied waking mind as the thought of the person coming — in a more free or in a concentrated state as a communication from the person in question; in a deeper concentration or in sleep or trance she would see the person coming and speaking to her or she herself going there. Besides that, wherever the Force is working, the Presence is there.

*

Mother's embodiment is a chance for the earth-consciousness to receive the Supramental into it and to undergo first the transformation necessary for that to be possible. Afterwards there will be a further transformation by the Supramental.

There is one divine Force which acts in the universe and in the individual and is also beyond the individual and the universe. The Mother stands for all these, but she is working here in the body to bring down something not yet expressed in this material world so as to transform life here — it is so that you should regard her as the Divine Shakti working here for that purpose. She is that in the body, but in her whole consciousness she is also identified with all the other aspects of the Divine.

*

The Divine Mother is the Consciousness and Force of the Divine — which is the Mother of all things.

It is the Divine who is the Master — the Self is inactive, it is always a silent witness supporting all things — that is the static aspect. There is also the dynamic aspect through which the Divine works — behind that is the Mother. You must not lose sight of that, that it is through the Mother that all things are attained.

*

The relation which exists between the Mother and all who accept her is a psychic and spiritual motherhood. It is a far greater relation than that of the physical mother to her child; it gives all that human motherhood can give, but in a much higher way, and it contains in itself infinitely more.

If the sadhak becomes unfaithful to the Mother, it means that he did not want the sadhana or the Mother but the satisfaction of his desires and his ego. That is not Yoga.

Mother has taken the body because a work of a physical nature (including a change in the physical world) had to be done. Some have come with her to share in the work, others she had called, others have come seeking for the light. With each she has a personal relation or a possibility of the personal relation, but each is of its own kind. To apply silly mathematical rules of the physical mind here is absurd. Your physical mind cannot understand what the Mother does, its values and standards and ideas are not hers. It is still worse to make your personal vital demand or desire the measure of what she ought to do. She acts in each case for different reasons suitable to that case.

Whether in work or in Yoga the Mother acts not from the mind or from the level of consciousness from which these criticisms arise, but from quite another vision and consciousness. If people want to understand why the Mother does things, let them get into the same inner consciousness from which she sees and acts. As to what she is, that also can only be seen either with the eye of faith or of a deeper vision.

*

It is the Purusha and Prakriti sides of the nature — one leading to pure conscious existence, static, the other to pure conscious force, dynamic — the Mother.

*

If I give, the Mother's force goes with it, or else the sadhak would get nothing, and if the Mother gives, my support goes with it and gives it my light as well as the Mother's. It is two sides of one indivisible action one carrying with it the other. It is the Mother's Force that gives the push.

*

The Mother's proposition is true. If one is open to Sri Aurobindo and not to the Mother it means that one is not really open to Sri Aurobindo. There is one force only, the Mother's force — or, if you like to put it like that, the Mother is Sri Aurobindo's Force.

*

This is what is termed the Adya Shakti; she is the Supreme Consciousness and Power above the universe and it is by her that all the Gods are manifested, and even the Supramental Ishwara comes into manifestation through her — the Supramental Purushottama of whom the Gods are Powers and Personalities.

*

As for the Mantra —, usually the Mother's name has the full power in it; but in certain states of consciousness the double Name [The Mother and Sri Aurobindo] may have a special effect.

*

A free and united India will be there and the Mother will gather around her sons and weld them into a single national strength in the life of a great and united people.

PROCESS OF SADHANA

There are two powers that alone can effect in their conjunction the great and difficult thing which is the aim of our endeavour, a fixed and unfailing aspiration that calls from below and a supreme Grace from above that answers.

But the supreme Grace will act only in the conditions of the Light and the Truth; it will not act in conditions laid upon it by the Falsehood and the Ignorance. For if it were to yield to the demands of the Falsehood, it would defeat its own purpose.

These are the conditions of the Light and Truth: —

There must be a total and sincere surrender; there must be an exclusive self-opening to the divine Power; there must be a constant and integral choice of the Truth that is descending, a constant and integral rejection of the falsehood of the mental, vital and physical Powers and Appearances that still rule the earth-Nature. The surrender must be total and seize all the parts of the being. There must be no part of the being, even the most external, anything that makes a reserve, anything that hides behind doubts, confusion and subterfuges, anything that revolts or refuses.

If behind your devotion and surrender you make a cover for your desires, egoistic demands and vital insistences, if you put these things in place of the true aspiration or mix them with it and try to impose them on the Divine Shakti, then it is idle to invoke the divine Grace to transform you. You must keep the temple clean if you wish to instal there the living Presence.

Reject the false notion that the divine Power will do and is bound to do everything for you at your demand and even though you do not satisfy the conditions laid down by the Supreme. Make your surrender true and complete, then only will all else be done for you. Reject too the false and indolent expectation that the divine Power will do even the surrender for you. The Supreme demands your surrender to her, but does not impose it; you are free at every moment, till the irrevocable transformation comes, to deny and to reject the Divine or to recall your self-giving, if you are willing to suffer the spiritual consequences. Your surrender must be self-made and free; it must be the surrender of a living being, not of an inert automaton or mechanical tool. A glad and strong and helpful submission is demanded to the working of the Divine Force, the obedience of the illumined disciple of the Truth, of the inner Warrior who fights against obscurity and falsehood, of the faithful servant of the Divine.

So long as the lower nature is active the personal effort of the sadhak remains necessary. The personal effort required is a triple labour of aspiration, rejection and surrender: —

(i) An aspiration vigilant, constant, unceasing.

(ii) Rejection of the movements of the lower nature.

(iii) Surrender of oneself and all one is and has.

In proportion as the surrender and self-consecration progress, the Sadhaka becomes conscious of the Divine Shakti doing the sadhana. The more this conscious process replaces his own effort, the more rapid and true becomes his progress. But it cannot completely replace the necessity of personal effort until the surrender and consecration are pure and complete from top to bottom. Note that a tamasic surrender refusing to fulfil the conditions and calling on God to do everything and save one all the trouble and struggle is a deception and does not lead to freedom and perfection....

To walk through life armoured against all fear, peril and disaster, only two things are needed, two that go always together — the Grace of the Divine Mother and on your side an inner state made up of faith, sincerity and surrender. Let your faith be pure, candid and perfect. An egoistic faith in the mental and vital being tainted by ambition, pride, vanity, mental arrogance, vital self-will, personal demand, desire for the petty satisfactions of the lower nature is a low and smoke-obscured flame that cannot burn upwards to heaven. Regard your life as given you only for the divine work and to help in the divine manifestation. Desire nothing but the purity, force, light, wideness, calm, Ananda of the divine consciousness and its insistence to transform and perfect your mind, life and body. Ask for nothing but the divine, spiritual and supramental Truth, its realisation on earth and in you and in all who are called and chosen and the conditions needed for its creation and its victory over all opposing forces.

Let your sincerity and surrender be genuine and entire. When you give yourself, give completely, without demand, without condition, without reservation so that all in you shall belong to the Divine Mother and nothing be left to the ego or given to any other power.

The more complete your faith, sincerity and surrender, the more will grace and protection be with you. And when the grace and protection of the Divine Mother are with you, what is there that can touch you or whom need you fear? A little of it even will carry you through all difficulties, obstacles and dangers; surrounded by its full presence you can go securely on your way because it is hers, careless of all menace, unaffected by any hostility however powerful, whether from this world or from worlds invisible. Its touch can turn difficulties into opportunities, failure into success and weakness into unfaltering strength.

*

While this transformation is being done it is more than ever necessary to keep yourself free from all taint of the perversions of the ego. Let no demand or insistence creep in to stain the purity of the self-giving and the sacrifice. There must be no attachment to the work or the result, no laying down of conditions, no claim to possess the Power that should possess you, no pride of the instrument, no vanity or arrogance. Nothing in the mind or in the vital or physical parts should be suffered to distort to its own use or seize for its own personal and separate satisfaction the greatness of the forces that are acting through you. Let your faith, your sincerity, your purity of aspiration be absolute and pervasive of all the planes and layers of the being; then every disturbing element and distorting influence will progressively fall away from your nature.

*

The sadhana of this Yoga does not proceed through any set mental teaching or prescribed forms of meditation, mantras or others, but by aspiration, by a self-concentration inwards or upwards, by self-opening to an Influence, to the Divine Power above us and its workings, to the Divine Presence in the heart and by the rejection of all that is foreign to these things. It is only by faith, aspiration and surrender that this self-opening can come.

*

It is not by taking a mere mental attitude that this can be done or even by any number of inner experiences which leave the outer man as he was. It is this outer man who has to open, to surrender and to change. His every least movement, habit, action has to be surrendered, seen, held up and exposed to the divine Light, offered to the divine Force for its old forms and motives to be destroyed and the divine Truth and the action of the transforming consciousness of the Divine Mother to take their place.

*

The constant presence of the Mother comes by practice; the Divine Grace is essential for success in the sadhana, but it is the practice that prepares the descent of the Grace.

You have to learn to go inward, ceasing to live in external things only, quiet the mind and aspire to become aware of the Mother's working in you.

*

Faith, reliance upon God, surrender and self-giving to the Divine Power are necessary and indispensable. But reliance upon God must not be made an excuse for indolence, weakness and surrender to the impulses of the lower Nature.

There is no method in this Yoga except to concentrate, preferably in the heart, and call the presence and power of the Mother to take up the being and by the workings of her force transform the consciousness. When the mind falls quiet and the concentration becomes strong and the aspiration intense, then there is a beginning of experience. The more the faith, the more rapid the result is likely to be. The bhakta does not rely on his own effort alone, but on the grace and power of the Divine whom he adores.

*

There are always difficulties and a hampered progress in the early stages and a delay in the opening of the inner doors until the being is ready. The road of Yoga is long, every inch of ground has to be won against much resistance and no quality is more needed by the sadhak than patience and single-minded perseverance with a faith that remains firm through all difficulties, delays and apparent failures.

Each part of the nature wants to go on with its old movements and refuses, so far as it can, to admit a radical change and progress, because that would subject it to something higher than itself and deprive it of its sovereignty in its own field, its separate empire. It is this that makes transformation so long and difficult a process.

The lower nature is ignorant and undivine, not in itself hostile but shut to the Light and Truth. The hostile forces are anti-divine, not merely undivine; they make use of the lower nature, pervert it, fill it with distorted movements and by that means influence man and even try to enter and possess or at least entirely contol him.

The rule in Yoga is not to let the depression depress you, to stand back from it, observe its cause and remove the cause. The Yogi should look on all the defects of the nature as movements of the lower prakriti common to all and reject them calmly, firmly and persistently with full confidence in the Divine Power. However hard the fight, the only thing is to fight it out now and here to the end.

*

The goal of Yoga is always hard to reach, but this one is more difficult than any other, and it is only for those who have the call, the capacity, the willingness to face everything and every risk, even the risk of failure, and the will to progress towards an entire selflessness, desirelessness and surrender.

*

All the ordinary vital movements are foreign to the true being and come from outside; they do not belong to the soul nor do they originate in it but are waves from the general Nature.

When one lives in the true consciousness one feels the desires outside oneself, entering from outside, from the universal lower Prakriti, into the mind and the vital parts.

Demand and desire are only two different aspects of the same thing. Demand or desire comes from the mental or the vital, but a psychic or spiritual need is a different thing. The psychic does not demand or desire — it aspires; it does not make conditions for its surrender or withdraw if its aspiration is not immediately satisfied — for the psychic has the complete trust in the Divine or in the Guru and can wait for the right time or the hour of the Divine Grace.

The supramental realisation is much more difficult and exacting in its conditions and the most difficult of all is to bring it down to the physical level.

You should not rely on anything else alone, however helpful it may seem, but chiefly, primarily, fundamentally on the Mother's Force. The sun and the Light may be a help but cannot take the place of the Mother's Force.

*

Our object is the supramental realisation and we have to do whatever is necessary for that or towards that under the conditions of each stage. At present the necessity is to prepare the physical consciousness; for that a complete equality and peace and a complete dedication free from personal demand or desire in the physical and the lower-vital parts are the things to be established. Other things can come in their proper time. What is needed now is the psychic opening in the physical consciousness and the constant presence and guidance there. It is this material consciousness into which we are seeking to bring first the higher Light and Power and Ananda, and then the Supramental Truth which is the object of our Yoga.

*

By remaining pschyically open to the Mother, all that is necessary for work or sadhana develops progressively, that is one of the chief secrets, the central secret of the sadhana.

To practice Yoga implies the will to overcome all attachments and turn to the Divine alone. The principal thing in the Yoga is to trust in the Divine Grace at every step, to direct the thought continually to the Divine and to offer oneself till the being opens and the Mother's force can be felt working in the Adhara.

To remain open to the Mother is to remain always quiet and

happy and confident — not restless, not grieving or despondent, to let her force work in you, guide you, give you knowledge, give you peace and Ananda.

It is by the constant remembrance that the being is prepared for the full opening. By the opening of the heart the Mother's presence begins to be felt and, by the opening to her Power above, the Force of the higher consciousness comes down into the body and works there to change the whole nature.

The direct opening of the psychic centre is easy only when the ego-centricity is greatly diminished and also if there is a strong bhakti for the Mother. A spiritual humility and sense of submission and dependence is necessary.

*

To be a Yogi, a Sannyasi, a Tapaswi is not the object here. The object is transformation, and the transformation can only be done by a force infinitely greater than your own; it can only be done by being truly like a child in the hands of the Divine Mother.

*

The effort demanded of the sadhak is that of aspiration, rejection and surrender. If these three are done the rest is to come of itself by the Grace of the Mother and the working of her Force in you. But of the three the most important is surrender of which the first necessary form is trust and confidence and patience in difficulty.

Nothing can be done except through the force of the Mother. All has to be done by the working of the Mother's force aided by your aspiration, devotion and surrender.

*

'X' is probably making two mistakes — first, expecting outward expressions of love from the Mother; second, looking for progress instead of concentrating on openness and surrender without demand of a return. These are two mistakes which sadhaks are constantly making. If one opens, if one surrenders, then as soon as the nature is ready, progress will come of itself; but the personal concentration for progress brings difficulties and resistance and disappointment because the mind is not looking at things from the right angle.

*

The sadhaks who enter the Yoga are human beings and if they were not allowed a human approach at the beginning and long after, they would not be able to start the Yoga or would not be able to continue it. But the human approach to the Divine should not be constantly turned into a human revolt and reproach against it.

*

The power needed in Yoga is the power to go through effort, difficulty or trouble without getting fatigued, depressed, discouraged or impatient and without breaking off the effort or giving up one's aim or resolution. A quiet vigilant but undistressed persistence is the best way to get the sadhana done.

*

It is because the vital is restless and full of desires that it is like that. Also the physical mind is by no means at rest. If the desires were thrown out and the ego less active and the physical mind at rest, knowledge would come from above in place of the physical mind's stupidities, the vital mind could be calm and quiet and the Mother's Force take up the action and the higher consciousness begin to come down.

*

The tendency to inquire and know is in itself good, but it must be kept under control. What is needed for progress in sadhana is gained best by increase of consciousness and experience and of intuitive knowledge.

*

The pressure and help of the Mother's Force is always there. Your rapidity of progress depends upon your keeping yourself open to it and rejecting calmly, quietly and steadily all suggestions and invasions of other forces. Especially the nervous excitement of the vital has to be rejected; a calm and quiet strength in the nervous being and the body is the only sound basis.

*

These are the main conditions of preparation for the supramental change, but none of them is easy, and they must be complete before the Adhara can be said to be ready. If the true attitude (psychic, unegoistic, open only to the Divine Force) can be established, then the process can go on much more quickly:—

1. Get the psychic being in the front and keep it there, putting its power on the mind, vital and physical, so that it shall communicate to them its force of single minded aspiration, trust, faith, surrender, direct and immediate detection of whatever is wrong in them and turned towards ego and error, away from Light and Truth.

2. Eliminate egoism in all its forms and from every movement of the consciousness.

3. Develop the cosmic consciousness — let the egocentric outlook disappear in wideness, impersonality, the sense of the cosmic divine, the perception of the universal force, the realisation and understanding of the cosmic manifestation, the play.

4. Find in place of ego the true being — a portion of the Divine, issued from the World-Mother and an instrument of the manifestation. This sense of being a portion of the Divine and an instru-

ment should be free from all pride, sense of claim of ego or assertion of superiority, demand or desire. For if these elements are there, then it is not the true thing.

5. Most in doing Yoga live in the mind, vital, physical, lit up occasionally or to some extent by the higher mind and by the illumined mind; but to prepare for the supramental change, it is necessary to open up to the intuition and the overmind, so that these may make the Adhara ready for the supramental change Allow the consciousness quietly to develop and widen and the knowledge of these things will progressively come.

6. Calm, discrimination, detachment (but not indifference) are all very important, for their opposites impede very much the transforming action. Intensity of aspiration should be there, but along with these, no hurry, no inertia — neither rajasik over-eagerness nor tamasic discouragement — a steady and persistent but quiet call and working. No snatching or clutching at realisation, but allowing realisation to come from within and above, and observing accurately its field, its nature, its limits.

7. Let the power of the Mother work in you, but be careful to avoid mixture or substitution in its place of either a magnified ego-working or a force of ignorance presenting itself as Truth. Aspire especially for the elimination of all obscurity and unconsciousness in the nature.

The Mother:

The question you are to answer is this: Do you want the Yoga for the sake of the Divine? Is the Divine the supreme fact of your life, so much so that it is simply impossible for you to do without it? Do you feel that your very *raison d'être* is the Divine and without it there is no meaning in your existence? If so, then only can it be said that you have a call for the path.

Aspiration for the Divine is the first thing necessary. The next thing you have to do is to tend it, to keep it always alert and awake and living. And for that what is required is concentration — concentration upon the Divine with a view to an integral and absolute consecration to its Will and Purpose.

Concentrate in the heart. Enter into it; go within and deep and far, as far as you can. Gather all the strings of your consciousness that are spread abroad, roll them up and take a plunge and sink down. A fire is burning there, in the deep quietude of the heart. It is the divinity in you — your true being. Hear its voice, follow its dictates.

To prepare oneself for the Yoga, one should be conscious, first of all. We are conscious of only an insignificant portion of our being; for the most part we are unconscious. It is this unconsciousness that keeps us tied down to our unregenerate nature and prevents change and transformation in it. It is through unconsciousness that the undivine forces enter into us and make us their slaves. You are to be conscious of yourself; that is to say, resolutely reject one and accept the other. The duality will present itself at every step and at every step you will have to make your choice. You will have to be patient and persistent and vigilant.

Yoga does become dangerous if you want it for your own sake, to serve a personal end. Dangers and difficulties come in when people take up Yoga, not for the sake of the Divine, but because they want to acquire power and under the guise of Yoga seek to satisfy some ambition. If you cannot get rid of ambition, do not touch the thing. It is fire that burns.

There are two paths of Yoga, one of *tapasyā* (discipline) and the other of surrender. The path of *tapasyā* is arduous, the path of surrender is safe and sure.

If you take up this path of surrender fully and sincerely, there is no more danger or serious difficulty. The question is to be sincere. If you are not sincere, do not begin Yoga. The first effect of Yoga, however, is to take away the mental control, and the hungers that lie dormant are suddenly set free, they rush up and invade the being. So long as this mental control has not been replaced by the Divine control, there is a period of transition when your sincerity and surrender will be put to test.

The impulses and desires that come up by the pressure of Yoga should be faced in a spirit of detachment and serenity, as something foreign to yourself or belonging to the outside world. They should be offered to the Divine, so that the Divine may take them up and transmute them.

If you have once opened your self to the Divine, if the power of the Divine has once come down into you and yet you try to keep to the old forces, you prepare troubles and difficulties and dangers for yourself. You must be vigilant and see that you do not use the Divine as a cloak for the satisfaction of your desires.

So long as you belong to humanity and so long as you lead the ordinary life, it does not matter much if you mix with the people of the world; but if you want the divine life, you will have to be exceedingly careful about your company and your environment. The whole world is full of the poison. You take it in with every breath. You can lose in a few minutes what it has taken you months to gain.

It is always wrong to display powers. This does not mean that there is no use for them. But they have to be used in the same way as they came. They come by union with the Divine. They must be used by the will of the Divine and not for display.

*

To enter the spiritual life means to take a plunge into the Divine, as you would jump into the sea. And that is not the end but the very beginning; for after you have taken the plunge, you must learn to live in the Divine. That is the plunge you have to take, and unless you do it, you may do Yoga for years and yet know nothing of a true spiritual living.

Yoga means union with the Divine, and the union is effected through offering — it is founded on the offering of yourself to the Divine. When the resolution has been taken, when you have decided that the whole of your life shall be given to the Divine, you have still at every moment to remember it and carry it out in all the details of your existence.

In the beginning of the Yoga you are apt to forget the Divine very often. But by constant aspiration you increase your remembrance and you diminish the forgetfulness. But this should not be done as a severe discipline or a duty; it must be a movement of love and joy.

SADHAK'S ATTITUDE

SUNLIT PATH :

The sunlit path can be followed by those who are able to practise surrender, first a central surrender and afterwards a more complete self-giving in all the parts of the being. If they can achieve and preserve the attitude of the central surrender, if they can rely wholly on the Divine and accept cheerfully whatever comes to them from the Divine, then their path becomes sunlit and may even be straightforward and easy. They will not escape all difficulties, no seeker can, but they will be able to meet them without pain and despondency....

The law is imposed on us by the Ignorance which is the nature of all our parts; our physical being is obviously a mass of ignorance, the vital is full of ignorant desires and passions, the mind is also an instrument of Ignorance struggling towards some kind of imperfect and mostly inferior and external knowledge. The path of the seeker proceeds through this ignorance; for a long time he can find no light of solid experience or realisation, only the hopes and ideas and beliefs of the mind which do not give the true spiritual seeing; or he gets glimpses of light or periods of light but the light often goes out and the luminous periods are followed by frequent or long periods of darkness....

If one has the faith or in the absence of faith the will to go through, one passes on and enters into the joy and light of the divine realisation. If one gets some habit of true surrender, then all this is not necessary; one can enter into the sunlit way....

The Purna Yoga means a fourfold path, a Yoga of Knowledge for the mind, a Yoga of Bhakti for the heart, a Yoga of works for the will and a Yoga of perfection for the whole nature....

The too great activity of the intellectual mind and its attachment to its own pride of ideas, its prejudices, its fixed notions and its ignorant reason may shut the doors to the inner light and prevent the full tide of Bhakti from flooding everything; it may also cling to a surface mental activity and refuse to go inside and allow the psychic vision and the feelings of the inner heart to become its guides, though it is by this vision and this feeling that Bhakti grows and conquers. So too the passions and desires of the vital being and its ego may block the way and prevent the self-giving of the mind and heart to the Divine....

One who is moved to Yoga by some curiosity of the mind or even by its desire for knowledge can turn aside from the path from disappointment or any other cause; still more can those who take it up from some inner ambition or vital desire turn away through revolt or frustration or the despondency of frequent check and failure....

Mind is our present topmost faculty; it is through the thinking mind and the heart with the soul, the psychic being behind them that we have to grow into the Spirit, for what the Force first tries to bring about is to fix the mind in the right central idea, faith or mental attitude and the right aspiration and poise of the heart and to make these sufficiently strong and firm to last in spite of other things in the mind and heart which are other than [they] or in conflict with them....

In any case, to begin with the vital is a hazardous affair; the difficulties there are more numerous and more violent than on the mental plane and the pitfalls are innumerable. The access to the soul, the psychic being is less easy because it is covered up with a thick veil of ego, passion and desire. One is apt to be swallowed up in a maze of vital experiences, not always reliable, the temptation of small siddhis, the appeal of the powers of darkness to the ego....

*

This Yoga demands a total dedication of the life to the aspiration for the discovery and embodiment of the Divine Truth and to nothing else whatsoever.

You must go inside yourself and enter into a complete dedication to the spiritual life. All clinging to mental preferences must fall away from you, all insistence on vital aims and interests and attachments must be put away, all egoistic clinging to family, friends, country must disappear if you want to succeed in Yoga.

The ways of the Divine are not like those of the human mind or according to our patterns and it is impossible to judge them or to lay down for Him what He shall or shall not do, for the Divine knows better than we can know. Not to impose one's mind and vital will on the Divine but to receive the Divine's will and follow it, is the true attitude of sadhana.

*

Fix upon your mind and heart the resolution to live for the Divine Truth and for that alone; reject all that is contrary and incompatible with it and turn away from the lower desires; aspire to open yourself to the Divine Power and to no other. Do this in all sincerity and the present and living help you need will not fail you.

The necessities of a sadhak should be as few as possible; for there are only a very few things that are real necessities in life. The rest are either utilities or things decorative to life or luxuries.

These, a Yogin has a right to possess or enjoy only on one of two conditions:

(a) if he uses them during his sadhana solely to train himself in possessing things without attachment or desire and learn to use them rightly, in harmony with the Divine Will, with a proper handling, a just organisation, arrangement and measure, —

(b) if he has already attained a true freedom from desire and attachment and is not in the least moved or affected in any way by loss or withholding or deprival. If he has any greed, desire, demand, claim for possession or enjoyment, any anxiety, grief, anger or vexation when denied or deprived, he is not free in spirit and his use of the things he possesses is contrary to the spirit of sadhana. Even if he is free in spirit, he will not be fit for possession if he has not learned to use things not for himself, but for the Divine Will, as an instrument, with the right knowledge and action in the use, for the proper equipment of a life lived not for oneself but for and in the Divine.

*

To remain within, above and untouched, full of the inner consciousness and the inner experience, — listening when need be to one or another with the surface consciousness, but with even that undisturbed, not either pulled outwards or invaded — that is the perfect condition for the sadhana.

*

Care should be taken that there should be no ambitious or selfish misuse, no pride or vanity, no sense of superiority, no claim or egoism of the instrument, only a simple and pure psychic instrumentation of the nature in any way in which it is fit for the service of the Divine.

Take with you the peace and quietude and joy and keep it by remembering always the Divine.

*

A mere restless dissatisfaction with the ordinary life is not a sufficient preparation for this Yoga. A positive inner call, a strong will and a great steadiness are necessary for success in the spiritual life.

*

Live always as if you were under the very eye of the Supreme and of the Divine Mother. Do nothing, try to think and feel nothing that would be unworthy of the Divine Presence.

*

It is not Yoga to give free play to the natural instincts and desires. Yoga demands mastery over the nature, not subjection to the nature.

It is the past habit of the vital that makes you repeatedly go out into the external part; you must persist and establish the opposite habit of living in your inner being which is your true being and of looking at everything from there. This Yoga is not of world-shunning asceticism, but of divine life.

*

Follow always the one rule, to open yourself directly to the Divine Force and not to others; if you keep in touch with it, all else will progressively arrange itself.

But in order that it may go on developing, you must become more quiet, more and more able to hold whatever comes without getting too eager and excited. Peace and calmness are the first thing — in the peace you can bear whatever love, Ananda, strength or knowledge comes.

*

Truth in speech and truth in thought are very important.

*

A spiritual atmosphere is more important than outer conditions; if one can get that and also create one's own spiritual air to breathe in and live in it, that is the true condition of progress.

*

The Mother is always near and within, it is only the obscurity of mind and vital that does not see or feel it. That is a knowledge which the mind of a sadhaka ought to hold firmly.

*

If a sadhak does anything wrong inwardly or outwardly, it creates a wrong influence in the atmosphere of the Ashram and opens the gates to the hostile Powers.

*

The feeling that all one does is from the Divine, that all action is the Mother's is a necessary step in experience, but one cannot remain in it — one has to go farther. Those can remain in it who do not want to change the nature but only to have experience of the Truth behind it.

One can be a conscious and perfect instrument only when one is no longer acting in obedience to the ignorant push of the lower nature but in surrender to the Mother and aware of her higher Force acting within oneself.

One must be vigilant, but not anxious and uneasy. The Mother's Force will act and bring the result in its own time, provided one offers all to her and aspires and is vigilant, calling and remembering her at all times, rejecting quietly all that stands in the way of the action of her transforming Force.

*

There should be not only a general attitude, but each work should be offered to the Mother so as to keep the attitude a living one all the time. There should be at the time of work no meditation, for that would withdraw the attention from the work, but there should be the constant memory of the One to whom you offer it. This is only a first process. When you begin to feel always that it is the Mother's force that is doing the work and you are only a channel or an instrument, then in place of memory there will have begun the automatic constant realisation of Yoga, divine union, in works.

*

Not only in your inward concentration, but in your outward acts and movements you must take the right attitude. If you do that and put everything under the Mother's guidance, you will find the difficulties begin to diminish or are much more easily got over and things become steadily smoother.

*

Demands should not be made; what you receive freely from the Mother helps you; what you demand or try to impose on her is bound to be empty of her force.

*

If vanity, ambition and self-conceit stand in your way, cast them from you. You will not get rid of these things by merely waiting for them to disappear. If you merely wait for things to happen, there is no reason why they should happen at all.

*

Once one has entered the path of Yoga, there is only one thing to do, to fix oneself in the resolution to go to the end whatever happens, whatever difficulties arise. None really gets the fulfilment in Yoga by his own capacity — it is by the greater Force that stands over you that it will come — and it is the call, persistent through all vicissitudes, to the Force, by which the fulfilment will come. Even when you cannot aspire actively, keep yourself turned to the Mother for the help to come — that is the one thing to do always.

*

Everyone who is turned to the Mother is doing my Yoga. It is a great mistake to suppose that one can "do" the Purna Yoga i.e. carry out and fulfil all the sides of the Yoga by one's own effort. No human being can do that. What one has to do is to put oneself in the Mother's hands and open oneself to her by service, by bhakti, by aspiration; then the Mother by her light and force works in him so that the sadhana is done. It is a mistake also to have the ambition to be a big Purna Yogi or a supramental being and ask oneself how far have I got towards that. The right attitude is to be devoted and given to the Mother and to wish to be whatever she wants you to be. The rest is for the Mother to decide and do in you.

*

There is one thing everybody should remember that everything should be done from the point of view of Yoga, of sadhana, of growing into a divine life in the Mother's consciousness. To insist upon one's own mind and its ideas, to allow oneself to be governed by one's own vital feelings and reactions should not be the rule of life here. One has to stand back from these, to be detached, to get in their place the true knowledge from above, the true feelings from the psychic within. This cannot be done if the mind and vital do not surrender, if they do not renounce their attachment to their own ignorance which they call truth, right, justice. All the trouble rises from that; if that were overcome, the basis of life, of work, of harmony, of all in the union with the Divine would more and more replace the trouble and difficulty of the present.

Our incapacity does not matter — there is no human being who is not in his parts of nature incapable — but the Divine Force is also there. If one puts one's trust in that, incapacity will be changed into capacity. Difficulties and struggles themselves then become a means towards the achievement.

It is when there is no attachment to outward things for their own sake and all is only for the Mother and the life through the inner psychic being is centred in her that the best condition is created for the spiritual realisation.

*

Those who are not straightforward cannot profit by the Mother's help, for they themselves turn it away. Unless they change, they cannot hope for the descent of the supramental Light and Truth into the lower vital and physical nature; they remain stuck in their own self-created mud and cannot progress.

*

One rule for you I can lay down, "Do not do, say or think anything which you would want to conceal from the Mother".

*

We must find the Self, the Divine, then only can we know what is the work the Self or the Divine demands from us. Until then our life and action can only be a help or means towards finding the Divine and it ought not to have any other purpose. But to decide beforehand by our limited mental conceptions what they must be is to hamper the growth of the spiritual Truth within.

The first necessity is the practice of concentration of your consciousness within yourself. The ordinary human mind has an activity on the surface which veils the real Self. But there is another, a hidden consciousness within behind the surface one in which we can become aware of the real Self and of a larger, deeper truth of nature, can realise the Self and liberate and transform the nature. To quiet the surface mind and begin to live within is the object of this concentration. To concentrate in the heart centre with the offering of oneself to the Divine and the aspiration for this inward opening and for the Presence in the heart is the first way and, if it can be done, the natural beginning; for its result once obtained makes the spiritual path far more easy and safe than if one begins the other way — but to begin with the heart centre, if one can do it, is the more desirable.

*

One must say "Since I want only the Divine, my success is sure, I have only to walk forward in all confidence and His own Hand will be there secretly leading me to Him by His own way and at His own time". That is what you must keep as your constant mantra.

*

As for the way out of the impasse you speak of, I know only of the quieting of the mind which makes meditation effective, purification of the heart which brings the Divine touch and in time the Divine Presence, humility before the Divine which liberates from egoism and pride of the mind and of the vital. What I have said is that you should not expect the Divine or insist on it at once or within an early time. It can come early or it can come late, but come it will if one is faithful in one's call.

*

Harmony and not strife is the law of yogic living. The aim here is fulfilment of the Divine in Life and for that, union and solidarity are indispensable. All jealousy, strife, hatred, aversion, rancour and other evil vital feelings should be abandoned as they can be no part of the spiritual life. So, also, all egoistic love and attachment will have to disappear — the love that loves only for the ego's sake and, as soon as the ego is hurt and dissatisfied, ceases to love or even cherishes rancour and hate. It is understood of course that such things as sexual impurity must disappear also.

*

The things that have to be established are: —

Brahmacharya, complete sex-purity; Shamah, quiet and harmony in the being, its forces maintained but controlled, harmonised, disciplined; Satyam, truth and sincerity in the whole nature; Prashantih, a general state of peace and calm; Atmasamyama, the power and habit to control whatever needs control in the movements of the nature. When these are fairly established, one has laid the foundation on which one can develop the Yoga consciousness and with the Yoga consciousness there comes an easy opening to realisation and experience. A Yoga like this needs patience, because it means a change both of the radical motives and of each part and detail of the nature.

*

Meditation is only a means or device, the true movement is when even walking, working and speaking, one is still in sadhana.

*

You must remain and grow always more and more deeply quiet and still both in yourself and in your attitude to the world around you. If you can do this, the sadhana is likely to go on progressing and enlarging itself with a minimum of trouble and disturbance.

You must gather yourself within more firmly. If you disperse yourself constantly, go out of the inner circle, you will constantly move about in the pettiness of the ordinary outer nature and under the influences to which it is open. Learn to live within, to act always from within, from a constant communion with the Mother. You must persist and establish the habit of living in your inner being which is your true being and of looking at everything from there.

*

The Mother's presence is always there; but if you decide to act on your own — your own idea, your own notion of things, your own will and demand upon things, then it is quite likely that her presence will get veiled; it is not she who withdraws from you, but you who draw back from her. But your mind and vital don't want to admit that, because it is always their preoccupation to justify their own movements. If the psychic were allowed its full predominance, this would not happen.

*

It is not advisable to cut oneself off from mixing with people altogether. You must remain in the higher consciousness even when with people.

*

Keep your aspiration strong and sincere and call in the Divine in each thing and at each moment for support and in all that you feel keep yourself open to us. That is the easiest way to the Divine.

*

Do not dwell much on the defect of others. It is not helpful. Keep always quiet and peace in the attitude.

*

Quarrels and clashes are a proof of the absence of the Yogic poise and those who seriously wish to do Yoga must learn to grow out of these things. It is easy enough not to clash when there is no cause for strife or dispute or quarrel; it is when there is cause and the other side is impossible and unreasonable that one gets the opportunity of rising above one's vital nature.

*

Efface the stamp of ego from the heart and let the love of the

Mother take its place. Cast from the mind all insistence on your personal ideas and judgement, then you will have the wisdom to understand her. Let there be no obsession of self-will, ego-drive in the action, love of personal authority, attachment to personal preference, then the Mother's force will be able to act clearly in you and you will get the inexhaustible energy for which you ask and your service will be perfect.

*

All should be done quietly from within — working, speaking, reading, writing as part of the real consciousness — not with the dispersed and unquiet movement of the ordinary consciousness. If you are troubled by failure or excited by success, that also you should overcome.

*

If one has the close inner relation, one feels the Mother always near and within and around and there is no insistence on the closer physical relation for its own sake .... If they get the outer closeness, they will find that it means nothing without the inner oneness and closeness. One may be physically near the Mother and yet will be as far from her as the Sahara desert.

*

If any sadhaka refuses in practice to admit this change or if he refuses even to admit the necessity for any change of his lower vital being and his habitual external personality, I am entitled to conclude that whatever his professions be has not accepted either myself or my Yoga.

Whatever the difficulties of the nature, however long and painful the process of dealing with them, they cannot stand to the end against the Truth, if there is or if there comes in these parts the true spirit, attitude and endeavour. But if a sadhaka continues out of self-esteem and self-will or out of tamasic inertia to shut his eyes or harden his heart against the Light, so long as he does that, no one can help him. The consent of all the being is necessary for the divine change, and it is the completeness and fullness of the consent that constitutes the integral surrender. But the consent of the lower vital must not be only a mental profession or a passing emotional adhesion; it must translate itself into an abiding attitude and a persistent and constant action.

*

There is a general protection around all the disciples, but most go out of it by their attitude, thoughts and actions or open the way to other forces.

*

To concentrate most on one's own spiritual growth and experience is the first necessity of the sadhak — to be eager to help others draws away from the inner work. To grow in the spirit is the greatest help one can give to others, for then something flows out naturally to those around that helps them.

*

Falsehood is a great barrier in the path of this Yoga. Falsehood of any kind must not be given a place in thought, speech or action.

The Mother:

When you come to the Divine, you must abandon all mental conceptions; but, instead of doing that, you throw your conceptions upon the Divine and want the Divine to obey them. The only true attitude for a Yogi is to be plastic and ready to obey the Divine command whatever it may be; nothing must be indispensable to him, nothing a burden. Often the first impulse of those who want to live the spiritual life is to throw away all they have; but they do it because they want to be rid of a burden, not because they want to surrender to the Divine. Men who possess wealth and are surrounded by the things that give them luxury and enjoyment turn to the Divine, and immediately their movement is to run away from these things and escape from their bondage. But it is a wrong movement; you must not think that the things you have belong to you, — they belong to the Divine. If the Divine wants you to enjoy anything, enjoy it; but be ready too to give it up the very next moment with a smile.

*

If we allow a falsehood, however small, to express itself through our mouth or our pen, how can we hope to become perfect messengers of Truth? A perfect servant of Truth should abstain even from the slightest inexactitude, exaggeration or deformation.

*

Do not worry about the reactions of people however unpleasant they may be — the vital is everywhere and in everybody full of impurities and the physical full of unconsciousness. These two imperfections have to be cured, however long it may take, and we have only to work at it patiently and courageously.

*

The force was acting chiefly in the mind, the vital and, through it, in the physical. It has come further down in its action and now it is at work not only in the material but also in the subconscient and even in the inconscient. Unless you follow this descending movement and allow the force to act in your body and the material regions of the consciousness, you will find yourself stranded on the road without being able to advance any further. And now to allow this working of the force, it is detailed surrender of all movements, habits, tastes, preferences, sense of necessities etc., that is urgently required.

*

He who wants to advance on the path of perfection must never complain of the difficulties on the way; for each one is an opportunity for a new progress. To complain is a sign of weakness and of insincerity.

*

The secret of this attainment of perfection lies in the sincere urge for it. In one's action one must be free from all social conventions, all moral prejudices. All physical activities should be organised entirely in such a way as to make the body grow in balance and force and beauty. With this end in view one must abstain from all pleasure-seeking including the sexual pleasure. For each sexual act is a step towards death.

*

Indeed one who wants to prepare for the supramental life should never allow his consciousness to slip down to dissipation and inconscience under the pretext of enjoyment or even rest and relaxation. The relaxation should be into force and light and not into darkness and weakness.

*

The two cannot go together; at every minute you have to decide whether you wish to remain within the manhood of yesterday or belong to the supermanhood of tomorrow. You must refuse to be moulded according to the life as it is and be successful in it, if you want to prepare for the life as it shall be and become its active and efficient member. You must deny yourself pleasures, if you wish to be open to the joy of living in integral beauty and harmony.

*

The senses should be able to bear everything without disgust or displeasure; at the same time they must acquire and develop more and more the power of discrimination with regard to the quality, origin and result of various vital vibrations and so know whether these are helpful to the poise and progress of the physical and vital being. Moreover, the senses should be utilised as instruments to approach and study the physical and vital worlds in all their complexities. Sensations are an excellent instrument for knowledge and education. To make them serve this purpose, they should not be used with an egoistic purpose, as a means of enjoyment, in a blind and ignorant seeking for pleasure and self-satisfaction.

It is by enlightening, strengthening and purifying the vital and not by weakening it that one can help towards the true progress of the being. To deprive oneself of sensations is as harmful as depriving oneself of food. But in the same way as the choice of food must be made with wisdom and only with a view to the growth and proper functioning of the body, the choice of sensations also should be made and control over them gained with a view only to the growth and perfection of this great dynamic instrument which is essential for the progress of all other parts of the being.

*

Yoga is not a joke; when you choose it you must know what you do. Once you have chosen it, you must stick to it. You have no right to waver, you must go through ....

To do this Yoga, the Yoga of transformation which is the most arduous, of all things, is possible only if you feel that you have come here for that — I mean here upon earth — that for you nothing else is worth doing, that this is the very reason of your existence. Even if you have to labour, suffer, struggle, it is of no importance; for you want that realisation and nothing else.

Once you have set your foot on the path of Yoga, you must have an iron resolution and walk straight to the goal at any cost ....

If you abandon the path, it is difficult even to find it again. What is strange is that if you leave it you lose it. There are legends to that effect in all countries, of people who abandoned the path and then have been seeking it again and have never regained it. It is as if it has vanished.

When you are on the path, do not leave it. Before you take it, hesitate, you may hesitate as long as you like. But as soon as you have taken it, it is finished, do not leave it any more; for that has consequences that may extend even to several lives. And that is extremely grave.

AIDS IN SADHANA

Aspiration

The aspiration must be intense, calm and strong but not restless and impatient, — then alone it can be stable.

You should aspire calmly — eat, sleep, do your work. Peace is the one thing you have to ask for now — it is only on the basis of peace and calm that the true progress and realisation can come. There must be no vital excitement in your seeking or your aspiration towards the Mother.

*

But why allow anything to come in the way between you and the Divine, any idea, any incident? When you are in full aspiration and joy, let nothing count, nothing be of any importance except the Divine and your aspiration. If one wants the Divine quickly, absolutely, entirely, that must be the spirit of approach, absolute, all-engrossing, making that the one point with which nothing else must interfere.

The Mother:

Grace is equally for all. But it is received according to the sincerity of each one. It does not depend on outward circumstances but on a sincere aspiration and openness.

Equanimity

Equality is the chief support of the true spiritual consciousness and it is this from which a Sadhaka deviates when he allows a vital movement to carry him away in feeling or speech or action. Equality means a quiet and unmoved mind and vital, it means not to be touched or disturbed by things that happen or things said or done to you, but to look at them with a straight look, free from the distortions created by personal feeling, and to try to understand what is behind them, why they happen, what is to be learnt from them, what is it in oneself which they are cast against and what inner profit or progress one can make out of them; it means self-mastery over the vital movements, — anger and sensitiveness and pride as well as desire and the rest, — not to let them get hold of the emotional being and disturb the inner peace, not to speak and act in the rush and impulsion of these things, always to act and speak out of a calm inner poise of the spirit.

The first condition of inner progress is to recognise whatever is or has been a wrong movement in any part of the nature, — wrong idea, wrong feeling, wrong speech, wrong action, — and by wrong is meant what departs from the truth, from the higher consciousness and higher self, from the way of the Divine.

Complete samata (equality) takes long to establish and it is dependent on three things — the soul's self-giving to the Divine by an inner surrender, the descent of the spiritual calm and peace from above and the steady long and persistent rejection of all egoistic, rajasic and other feelings that contradict samata.

*

There can be no firm foundation in sadhana without equality. Whatever the unpleasantness of circumstances, however disagreeable the conduct of others, you must learn to receive them with a perfect calm and without any disturbing reaction. These things are the test of equality. It is easy to be calm and equal when things go well and people and circumstances are pleasant; it is when they are the opposite that the completeness of the calm, peace, equality can be tested, reinforced, made perfect.

*

No doubt, hatred and cursing are not the proper attitude. It is true also that to look upon all things and all people with a calm and clear vision, to be uninvolved and impartial in one's judgements is a quite proper Yogic attitude. A condition of perfect samata can be established in which one sees all as equal, friends and enemies included, and is not disturbed by what men do or by what happens.

*

Equanimity and peace in all conditions, in all parts of the being is the first foundation of the Yogic status. Peace is the first condition without which nothing else can be stable.

*

Equality means another thing — to have an equal view of men and their nature and acts and the forces that move them; it helps one to see the Truth about them by pushing away from the mind all personal feeling in one's seeing and judgement and even all mental bias. For a sadhak, to live rather in the calm strength of the spirit is an essential part of his progress.

The Mother:

You must have a strong body and strong nerves. You must have a strong basis of equanimity in your external being. Equanimity is the essential condition of union and communion with the Divine. If you have this basis, you can contain a world of emotion and yet not have to scream it out. This does not mean that you cannot express your emotion, but you can express it in a beautiful, harmonious way. To weep or scream or dance about with the descent of some kind of higher joy or experience is always a proof of weakness, either of the vital or the mental or the physical nature. If you have to bear the pressure of the Divine descent, you must be very strong and powerful, otherwise you would be shaken to pieces. If a little drop makes you sing and dance and scream, what would happen if the whole thing came down?

*

All feelings of shrinking and disgust and fear that disturb and weaken the human mind can be overcome. A Yogi has to overcome these reactions; for almost the very first step in Yoga demands that you must keep a perfect equanimity in the presence of all beings and things and happenings. Always you must remain calm, untouched and unmoved; the strength of the Yogi lies there. An entire calmness and quietness will disarm even dangerous and ferocious animals when they confront you.

*

Keep a cheerful mind and a peaceful heart. Let nothing disturb your equanimity and make every day the necessary progress to advance with me steadily towards the goal.

Faith

The phrase "Blind faith" has no real meaning. I suppose they mean they will not believe without proof — but the conclusion formed after proof is not faith, it is knowledge or it is a mental opinion. Faith is something which one has before proof or knowledge and it helps you to arrive at knowledge or experience. There is no proof that God exists, but if I have faith in God, then I can arrive at the experience of the Divine.

There are four kinds of faith: Mental faith combats doubts and helps to open to the true knowledge; vital faith prevents the attacks of the hostile forces or defeats them and helps to open to the true spiritual will and action; physical faith keeps one firm through all physical obscurity, inertia or suffering and helps to open to the foundation of the true consciousness; psychic faith opens to the direct touch of the Divine and helps to bring union and surrender.

*

Faith can be tamasic and ineffective, i.e., "I believe the Mother will do everything, so I will do nothing. When she wants, she will transform me." That is not a dynamic but a static and inert faith.

*

The faith in spiritual things that is asked of the sadhak is not an ignorant but a luminous faith, a faith in light and not in darkness. It is called blind by the sceptical intellect because it refuses to be guided by outer appearances or seeming facts.

Faith does not depend upon experience; it is something that is there before experience. When one starts the Yoga, it is not usually on the strength of experience, but on the strength of faith. It is so not only in Yoga and the spiritual life, but in ordinary life also. All men of action, discoverers, inventors, creators of knowledge proceed by faith and, until the proof is made or the thing done, they go on in spite of disappointment, failure, disproof, denial because of something in them that tells them that this is the truth, the thing that must be followed and done....

*

Faith is a certitude in the soul which does not depend on reasoning, on this or that mental idea, on circumstances, on this or that passing condition of the mind or the vital or the body.

The Mother:

No attachments, no desires, no impulses, no preferences; perfect equanimity, unchanging peace and absolute faith in the Divine protection, with that you are safe, without it you are in peril. And as long as you are not safe, it is better to do like little chickens that take shelter under the Mother's wings.

*

It is in proportion to our trust in the Divine that the Divine Grace can act for us and help.

*

If you keep your faith unshaken and your heart always open to me then all difficulties, however great, will contribute to the greater perfection of your being.

*

For nobody sadhana would be possible without the Divine's help. The Grace is always there ready to act but you must let it work and not resist its action. The one condition required is faith. When you feel attacked call for help to Sri Aurobindo and myself.

If your call is sincere it will be answered and the Grace will cure you.

*

A faith based on material proofs is not faith — it is a bargaining.

*

Never forget that you are not alone. The Divine is with you helping and guiding you. He is the companion who never fails, the friend whose love comforts and strengthens. Have faith and He will do everything for you.

Guru:

Up to now no liberated man has objected to the Guruvada; it is usually only people who live in the mind or vital and have the pride of the mind and the arrogance of the vital that find it below their dignity to recognise a Guru.

*

A human soul and nature cannot be dealt with by a set of mental rules applicable to everybody in the same way; if it were so, there would be no need of a Guru, each could set his chart of Yogic rules before him like the rules of Sandow's exercise and follow them till he becomes the perfect Siddha!

*

Because all Gurus are the same Divine, it does not follow that the disciple does well if he leaves the one meant for him to follow another. Fidelity to the Guru is demanded of every disciple.

*

From a humbug you can get nothing but his humbuggery. He must have something in him which makes the contact with the Divine possible, something which works even if he is not in his outer mind quite conscious of its action. If there is nothing at all spiritual in him, he is not a Guru, only a pseudo.

*

Many people have a habit of doing Yoga according to their own ideas without caring for the guidance of a Guru — from whom, however, they expect an entire protection and success in sadhana even if they prance or gambol into the wrongest paths possible.

*

Each man who enters the realms of yogic experience is free to follow his own way; but this yoga is not a path for anyone to follow, but only for those who accept to seek the aim, pursue the way pointed out upon which a sure guidance is indispensable. It is idle for anyone to expect that he can follow this road far, — much less go to the end by his own inner strength and knowledge without the true aid or influence. Even the ordinary long-practised yogas are hard to follow without the aid of the Guru; in this which as it advances goes through untrodden countries and unknown entangled regions, it is quite impossible.

The Mother:

Be faithful to your Guru whoever he is, he will lead you as far as you can go.

But if you are lucky enough to have the Divine as your Guru then there will be no limit to your realisation.

Meditation and Concentration

There is no harm in concentrating sometimes in the heart and sometimes above the head. But concentration in either place does not mean keeping the attention fixed on a particular spot; you have to take your station of consciousness in either place and concentrate there not on the place, but on the Divine. This can be done with eyes shut or with eyes open, according as best suits you.

In this Yoga the whole principle is to open oneself to the Divine Influence. It is there above you and, if you can once become conscious of it, you have then to call it down into you. It descends into the mind and into the body as Peace, as a Light, as a Force that works, as the Presence of the Divine with or without form, as Ananda. Before one has this consciousness, one has to have faith and aspire for the opening. Aspiration, call, prayer are forms of one and the same thing and are all effective; you can take the form that comes to you or is easiest to you. The other way is concentration; you concentrate your consciousness in the heart and meditate on the Mother in the heart and call her in there. One can do either and both at different times — whatever comes naturally to you or you are moved to do at the moment. Especially in the beginning the one great necessity is to get the mind quiet, reject at the time of meditation all thoughts and movements that are foreign to the sadhana. In the quiet mind there will be a progressive preparation for the experience. But you must not become impatient, if all is not done at once; it takes time to bring entire quiet into the mind; you have to go on till the consciousness is ready.

*

As a rule the only mantra used in this sadhana is that of the Mother or of my name and the Mother's. The concentration in the heart and the concentration in the head can both be used — each has its own result.

There is no method in this Yoga except to concentrate, preferably in the heart, and call the presence and power of the Mother to take up the being and by the workings of her force transform the consciousness. When the mind falls quiet and the concentration becomes strong and the aspiration intense, then there is a beginning of experience. The more the faith, the more rapid the result is likely to be.

*

When one tries to meditate, there is pressure to go inside, lose the waking consciousness and wake inside, in a deep inner consciousness. But at first the mind takes it for a pressure to go to sleep, since sleep is the only kind of inner consciousness to which it has been accustomed. In Yoga by meditation sleep is therefore often the first difficulty — but if one perseveres, then gradually the sleep changes to an inner conscious state.

*

There is no necessity of losing consciousness when you meditate. It is the widening and change of the consciousness that is essential.

*

In order to have Dhyana, the restlessness of the mind must be utterly settled, the intellect must become like a calm and waveless sea, not a ripple on its surface. The distinguishing feature of Dhyana is that it puts out a steady force of knowledge on the object of knowledge.

*

Concentration is a gathering together of the consciousness and either centralising at one point or turning on a single object, e.g., the Divine; there can also be a gathered condition throughout the whole being, not at a point. In meditation it is not indispensable to gather like this, one can simply remain with a quiet mind thinking of one subject or observing what comes in the consciousness and dealing with it....

Concentration means fixing the consciousness in one place or on one object and in a single condition. Meditation can be diffusive, e.g., thinking about the Divine, receiving impressions and discriminating, watching what goes on in the nature and acting upon it etc.

The best help for concentration is to receive the Mother's calm and peace into your mind. It is there above you — only the mind and its centres have to open to it....

It is to remain quiet at the time of meditation, not fighting with the mind or making mental efforts to pull down the Power or the Silence but keeping only a silent will and aspiration for them. If the mind is active, one has to learn to look at it, draw back and not giving any sanction from within, until its habitual or mechanical activities begin to fall quiet for want of support from within. If it is too persistent, a steady rejection without strain or struggle is the one thing to be done.

*

The two main places where one can centre the consciousness for Yoga are in the head and in the heart. The sitting motionless posture is the natural posture for concentrated meditation — walking and standing are active conditions. One can accustom oneself to meditate walking, standing, lying but sitting is the first natural position.

It is better to make the deeper concentration when you are alone or quiet. Outward sounds ought not to disturb you. The concentration is in its nature quiet and steady. If there is restlessness or over-eagerness, then that is not concentration.

There are always two things that can rise up and assail the silence, — vital suggestions, the physical mind's mechanical recurrences. Calm rejection for both is the cure. One can remain separate and see the thoughts and imaginations pass without being affected, but that is not being plunged or engrossed in meditation.

*

You have asked what is the discipline to be followed in order to convert the mental seeking into a living spiritual experience. The first necessity is the practice of concentration of your consciousness within yourself. The ordinary human mind has an activity on the surface which veils the real self. But there is another, a hidden consciousness within behind the surface one in which we can become aware of the real self and of a larger deeper truth of nature, can realise the self and liberate and transform the nature. To quiet the surface mind and begin to live within is the object of this concentration. Of this true consciousness other than the superficial there are two main centres, one in the heart (not the physical heart but the cardiac centre in the middle of the chest,) one in the head. The concentration in the heart opens within and by following this inward opening and going deep one becomes aware of the soul or psychic being, the divine element in the individual. This being unveiled begins to come forward, to govern the nature, to turn it and all its movements towards the Truth, towards the Divine, and to call down into it all that is above. It brings the consciousness of the Presence, the dedication of the being to the Highest and invites the descent into our nature of a greater Force and Consciousness which is waiting above us. To concentrate in the heart centre with the offering of oneself to the Divine and the aspiration for this inward opening and for the Presence in the heart is the first way and, if it can be done, the natural beginning; for its result once obtained makes the spiritual path far more easy and safe than if one begins the other way....

Finally, in all difficulties where personal effort is hampered the help of the Teacher can intervene and bring about what is needed for the realisation or for the immediate step that is necessary.

*

Concentration is necessary, first, to turn the whole will and mind from the discursive divagation natural to them, following a dispersed movement of the thoughts, running after many-branching desires, led away in the track of the senses and the outward mental response to phenomena: we have to fix the will and the thought on the eternal and real behind all, and this demands an immense effort, a one-pointed concentration. Secondly, it is necessary in order to break down the veil which is erected by our ordinary mentality between ourselves and the truth; for our knowledge can be picked up by the way, by ordinary attention and reception, but the inner, hidden and higher truth can only be seized by an absolute concentration of the mind on its object, an absolute concentration of the will to attain it and, once attained, to hold it habitually and securely unite oneself with it.

The Mother:

The number of hours spent in meditation is no proof of spiritual progress. It is a proof of your progress when you no longer have to make an effort to meditate. Then you have rather to make an effort to stop meditation: it becomes difficult to stop meditation, difficult to stop thinking of the Divine, difficult to come down to the ordinary consciousness. Then you are sure of your progress, then you have made real progress when concentration in the Divine is the necessity of your life, when you cannot do without it, when it continues naturally from morning to night, whatever you may be engaged in doing. What is required of you is consciousness; to be constantly conscious of the Divine. If you need to make an effort to go into meditation, you are still very far from being able to live the spiritual life. The final aim is to be in constant union with the Divine, not only in meditation but in all circumstances and in all the active life.

*

Collective meditation is not desirable. I do not approve of it. It brings more troubles. It is not safe, so it is better that it is dropped....

Yes, if one has to say something or tell or talk or to read something from the Mother or Sri Aurobindo or somebody explains the works of Sri Aurobindo and the Mother, it is all right that you meet together and remain together, but not to meditate.

The meditation can be collective and it is very good and it energises a great force, but it is only when the members who collect together for the meditation are single-minded, in full harmony and co-operation, they are together for one single ideal, one and not divided — all as one block or one single unit. That too not many but a selected few. It is most important to have an inner vision and discrimination in choosing people for meditation.

*

It is a meditation which has the power to transform your being, a meditation which is progressive. Usually people do not have a dynamic meditation. When they enter into what they call meditation, it is a kind of immobility in which nothing changes; they come out of it just as they entered into it, without any progress either in their being or in their consciousness. They could meditate in this way for eternities and it would bring no change either in themselves or in the universe. That is why Sri Aurobindo speaks of dynamic meditation, for it is just the contrary: it is transforming meditation.

*

It is always better to concentrate in one centre, preferably the centre of aspiration, the place where the flame burns; bring all the energies there, in the centre of the solar plexus, and if possible secure an attentive silence as if you wanted to listen to something extremely subtle, something that needs an entire attention, a complete concentration and a total Silence, and then move no more. No more thinking, no more moving but laying yourself open so as to receive all that can be received, taking care at the same time not to try to know what is happening at the moment when it is happening; for if you want to understand or even to observe actively, that keeps on a kind of cerebral activity which is unfavourable to the fullness of the receptivity. Therefore keep silent, as completely silent as possible, in an attentive concentration and then remain immobile.

Peace

The first thing to do in the sadhana is to get a settled peace and silence in the mind. Otherwise you may have experiences, but nothing will be permanent. It is in the silent mind that the true consciousness can be built....

The forces that stand in the way of sadhana are the forces of the lower mental, vital and physical nature. Behind them are adverse powers of the mental, vital and subtle physical worlds. These can be dealt with only after the mind and heart have become one-pointed and concentrated in the single aspiration to the Divine....

Aspire to the Mother for this settled quietness and calm of the mind and this constant sense of the inner being in you standing back from the external nature and turned to the Light and Truth....

The important thing is to get rid of the habit of the invasion of troubling thoughts, wrong feelings, confusion of ideas, unhappy movements. These disturb the nature and cloud it and make it difficult for the Force to work; when the mind is quiet and at peace, the Force can work more easily.

*

Aspire for the rest of the divine consciousness, but with a calm and deep aspiration. It can be ardent as well as calm, but not impatient, restless or full of rajasic eagerness. Remain quiet, open yourself and call the divine Shakti to confirm the calm and peace, to widen the consciousness and to bring into it as much light and power as it can receive and assimilate. Take care not to be over-eager, as this may disturb such quiet and balance as has been already established in the vital nature.

*

To remain quiet within, firm in the will to go through, refusing to be disturbed or discouraged by difficulties or fluctuations, that is one of the first things to be learned in the path.

*

Here as elsewhere, quiet is the first thing needed, to keep the consciousness quiet, not allow it to get agitated and in turmoil. Then in the quiet to call for the Force to clear up all this obscurity and change it.

*

To develop in the physical itself a constant will for the drawing down of the higher consciousness — especially the Peace and Force from above, is the best way out of it.

*

The one thing that is most needed for this sadhana is peace, calm, especially in the vital — a peace which depends not on circumstances or surroundings but on the inner contact with a higher consciousness which is the consciousness of the Divine, of the Mother. Those who have not that or do not aspire to get it can come here and live in the Ashram for ten or twenty years and yet be as restless and full of struggle as ever, — those who open their minds and vital to the Mother's strength and peace get it even in the hardest and most unpleasant work and the worst circumstances.

*

A quiet mind and a quiet vital are the first conditions for success in sadhana.

*

You must make grow in you the peace that is born of the certitude of victory.

The Mother:

The Divine Consciousness is at work to transform you and you must open to it in order to let it work freely in you. Be quiet always, calm, peaceful and let the Force work in your consciousness through the transparency of a perfect sincerity.

It is only in quietness and peace that one can know what is the best thing to do.

*

Establish a greater peace and quietness in your body, that will give you the strength to resist attacks of illness.

*

Increase the inner rest, it must become a rest always present even in the midst of the greatest activity and so steady that nothing has the power to shake it — and then you will become a perfect instrument for the Manifestation.

*

Be very careful to remain always calm and peaceful and let an integral equanimity establish itself more and more completely in your being. Do not allow your mind to be too active and to live in a turmoil, do not jump to conclusions from a superficial view of things; always take your time, concentrate and decide only in quietness.

*

Be quiet and gather strength and force not only to do work but also chiefly to achieve the Transformation.

Personal Effort

Personal effort is needed for opening yourself more and more by assent to the true things, Peace, Light, Truth, Ananda — by refusing the wrong things, such as anger, falsehood, lust etc.

*

It is the wrong movements, — self-will, egoism, the vital passions, vanity, personal desires etc. that stand in the way of giving full assent to the Mother's working in the sadhak's nature.

*

If there is no personal effort, if the sadhak is too indolent and tamasic to try, why should the Grace act?

*

Note that a tamasic surrender refusing to fulfil the conditions and calling on God to do everything and save one all the trouble and struggle is a deception and does not lead to freedom and perfection.

*

So long as there is not the full Presence and conscious working of the higher Force, some amount of the personal effort is indispensable. To do the sadhana for the sake of the Divine and not for one's own sake is of course the true attitude.

Psychic Being

The soul, the psychic being is in direct touch with the Divine Truth, but it is hidden in man by the mind, the vital being and the physical nature. If there is a refusal of the psychic new birth, a refusal to become the child new born from the Mother, owing to attachment to intellectual knowledge or mental ideas or to some vital desire, then there will be a failure in the sadhana.

*

If you want a more swift and visible progress, it can only be by bringing your psychic to the front through a constant self-offering. Aspire intensely, but without impatience.

*

The psychic being will not need the support of intellectual ideas or outer signs and helps. It is that alone that can give you the direct feeling of the Divine, the constant nearness, the inner support and aid. You will not then feel the Mother remote or have any further doubt about the realisation; for the mind thinks and the vital craves, but the soul feels and knows the Divine. If you want to succeed in this Yoga, you must take your stand on the psychic relation and reject the egoistic vital movement. The psychic being coming to the front and staying there is the decisive movement in the Yoga.

*

Happiness comes from the soul's satisfaction, not from the vital's or the body's. The vital is never satisfied; the body soon ceases to be moved at all by what it easily or always has. Only the psychic being brings the real joy and felicity.

*

Aspiration, constant and sincere, and the will to turn to the Divine alone are the best means to bring forward the psychic.

*

Purification and consecration are two great necessities of sadhana. Those who have experiences before purification run a great risk: it is much better to have the heart pure first, for then the way becomes safe. That is why I advocate the psychic change of the nature first — for that means the purification of the heart.

*

The psychic being is a portion of the Divine; it has a natural attraction for the Truth and the Divine but that attraction is desireless, free from demands and lower cravings.

*

Awakening means the conscious action of the psychic from behind. When psychic comes to the front, it invades the mind and vital and body and psychicises their movements. It comes best by aspiration and an unquestioning and entire turning and surrender to the Mother.

*

The inner being is composed of the inner mental, the inner vital, the inner physical. The psychic is the inmost supporting all the others.

*

It is the soul, the psychic being in you, behind the heart, that is awake and wants to concentrate the mind on the Divine. It is the nature of the mind to go out to other things, but now when it does that there is the unease in the heart, the psychic sorrow, because the heart feels at once that this is wrong and the head also aches because of the resistance to the Divine Force at work. This is a thing that often happens at an early stage, after the opening of the consciousness to the sadhana.

*

The psychic being is one's own individual soul-being. It is not the Divine, though it has come from the Divine and develops towards the Divine.

The Mother:

There is not one person in a million who has a conscious relation with his psychic being, even for a moment. The psychic being can work from within, but, for the external being, in such an invisible and unconscious way as if it did not exist. In most cases, in almost all cases, in fact, the psychic being is asleep, as it were, not active at all, but in a kind of torpor. It is only by Sadhana and persistent effort that one can arrive at a conscious connection with one's psychic being.

*

I am always present in your psychic being. It is there that you can and ought to find me, and when you will find me there, in the depths of your heart, you will recognise me also in my physical form.

SILENCE

The silent mind is a result of Yoga; the ordinary mind is never silent.

Mother does not approve at all of the idea of a complete retirement. It does not bring the control — it is a control established while in contact with the outward things that is alone genuine. You must establish that from within by a fixed resolution and practice. Too much mixing and too much talk should be avoided, but a complete retirement is not the thing. It has not had the required result with anyone so far.

The Mother:

It is only in silence that a true progress can be made; it is only in silence that one can rectify a wrong movement; it is only in silence that one can be of help to somebody else.

SINCERITY

To be entirely sincere means to desire the divine Truth only, to surrender yourself more and more to the Divine Mother, to reject all personal demand and desire other than this one aspiration, to offer every action in life to the Divine and do it as the work given without bringing in the ego. This is the basis of the divine life.

*

You have only to be perfectly sincere and aspire for purification and reject whatever is wrong in you. The Divine Force will then act and do the rest. That is the simple and true way.

*

The house of the Divine is not closed to any who knock sincerely at its gates, whatever their past stumbles and errors.

*

A greater power is sincerity; a greatest power of all is Grace.

*

The Divine gives the fruit not by the measure of the sadhana but by the measure of the soul's sincerity and its aspiration. One should say: "I am ready to be not what I want but what the Divine wants me to be".

*

Open with sincerity. That means to open integrally and without reservation; not to give one part of you to the divine working and keep back the rest; not to make a partial offering and keep for yourself the other movements of your nature. All must be opened wide; it is insincerity to hold back any part of you or keep it shut to the Divine.

Open with faithfulness. That means to be open constantly and always; not to open one day and withdraw the next.

The Mother:

In order to be always near me really and effectively you must become more and more sincere, open and frank towards me.

*

Sincerity is the key of the divine doors.

*

As long as there is within the being the possibility of an inner conflict it means that there is still in him some insincerity.

Surrender

A complete surrender is not possible in so short a time, — for a complete surrender means to cut the knot of the ego in each part of the being and offer it, free and whole, to the Divine.

*

It is not possible to get rid of the stress on personal effort at once — and not always desirable; for personal effort is better than tamasic inertia. The personal effort has to be transformed progressively into a movement of the Divine Force.

It is not advisable in the early stages of the sadhana to leave everything to the Divine or expect everything from it without the need of one's own endeavour. That is only possible when the psychic being is in front. Under other conditions this attitude is likely to lead to stagnation and inertia.

It is ego and desire that prevent surrender. If there is no surrender, there can be no transformation of the whole being. Absolute sincerity can make the determination of surrender rapidly effective.

*

Active surrender is when you associate your will with the Divine Will, reject what is not the Divine, assent to what is the Divine. Passive surrender is when everything is left entirely to the Divine — it turns out that you surrender to the lower nature under pretext of surrendering to the Divine.

*

True surrender is possible when the sadhak is able to get rid of these things — accept the knowledge from above in place of his own ideas, the will of the Divine in place of his own desires, the movements of the Truth in place of his physical habits — and as a result is able to live wholly for the Divine.

*

Self-giving or surrender is demanded of those who practise this Yoga, because without such a progressive surrender of the being it is quite impossible to get anywhere near the goal. To keep open means to call in Mother's Force to work in you, and if you do not surrender to it, it amounts to not allowing the Force to work in you at all or else only on condition that it will work in the way you want and not in its own way which is the way of the Divine Truth.

*

It is necessary if you want to progress in your sadhana that you should make the submission and surrender of which you speak sincere, real and possible. This cannot be as long as you mix up your desires with your spiritual aspiration. It cannot be as long as you cherish vital attachment to family, child or anything or anybody else. If you are to do this Yoga, you must have only one desire and aspiration, to receive the spiritual Truth and manifest it in all your thoughts, feelings, actions and nature. You must not hunger after any relations with anyone.

*

To give oneself is the secret of sadhana, not to demand and acquire a thing. The more one gives oneself, the more the power to receive will grow. But for that all impatience and revolt must go; all suggestions of not getting, not being helped, not being loved, going away, of abandoning life or the spiritual endeavour must be rejected.

*

The whole principle of this Yoga is to give oneself entirely to the Divine alone and to nobody and nothing else, and to bring down into ourselves by union with the Divine Mother-Power all the transcendent light, force, wideness, peace, purity, truth-consciousness and Ananda of the supramental Divine. In this Yoga, therefore, there can be no place for vital relations or interchanges with others; any such relation or interchange immediately ties down the soul to the lower consciouness and its lower nature, prevents the true and full union with the Divine and hampers both the ascent to the supramental Truth-Consciousness and the descent of the supramental Ishwari Shakti.

*

There is no single rule for all, it depends on the personality and the nature. Surrender is the main power of the Yoga, but the surrender is bound to be progressive; a complete surrender is not possible in the beginning, but only a will in the being for that completeness. It is only when the surrender is complete that the full flood of sadhana is possible. Till then there must be the personal effort with an increasing reality of surrender.

*

It is altogether unprofitable to enquire who or what class will arrive first or last at the goal. The spiritual path is not a field of competition or a race that this should matter. What matters is one's own aspiration for the Divine, one's own faith, surrender, selfless self-giving. Others can be left to the Divine who will lead each according to his nature. Meditation, work, bhakti are each means of preparative help towards fulfilment; all are included in this path. If one can dedicate oneself through work, that is one of the most powerful means towards the self-giving which is itself the most powerful and indispensable element of the sadhana.

*

The true movement is a pure aspiration and surrender. After all, one has not a right to call on the Divine to manifest himself; it can come only as a response to a spiritual or psychic state of consciousness or to a long course of sadhana rightly done; or, if it comes before that or without any apparent reason, it is a Grace; but one cannot demand or compel Grace. Grace is something spontaneous which wells out from the Divine Consciousness as a free flow of its being. The bhakta looks for it, but he is ready to wait in perfect reliance — even if need be, all his life — knowing that it will come, never varying in his love and surrender because it does not come now or soon.

*

It is the first principle of our sadhana that surrender is the means of fulfilment and so long as ego or vital demand and desire are cherished, complete surrender is impossible. You have to go on rejecting the vital mixture everytime it rises. If you are steadfast in rejecting, it will lose more and more of its force and fade out.

Always keep within and do things without involving yourself in them, then nothing adverse will happen or, if it does, no serious reaction will come.

Self-surrender to the divine and infinite Mother, however difficult, remains our only effective means and our sole abiding refuge, — self-surrender to her means that our nature must be an instrument in her hands, the soul a child in the arms of the Mother.

*

This Yoga accepts the value of cosmic existence and holds it to be a reality; its object is to enter into a higher Truth-Consciousness or Divine Supramental Consciousness in which action and creation are the expression not of ignorance and imperfection, but of the Truth, the Light, the Divine Ananda. But for that, surrender of the mortal mind, life and body to that Higher Consciousness is indispensable, since it is too difficult for the mortal human being to pass by its own effort beyond mind to a Supramental Consciousness in which the dynamism is no longer mental but of quite another power. Only those who can accept the call to such a change should enter into this Yoga.

The Mother:

In our Yoga there is no room for sacrifice. In its pure sense it means a consecrated giving, a making sacred to the Divine.... If you have the slightest feeling that you are making sacrifice, then it is no longer surrender.... True surrender enlarges you; it increases your capacity; it gives you a greater measure in quality and in quantity, which you could not have had by yourself.

*

Give all you are, all you have, nothing more is asked of you but also nothing less.

*

Even the gods have to make their surrender to the Supreme, if the Divine creation is to be realised upon the earth.

*

The true, lasting quietness in the vital and the physical as well as in the mind, comes from a complete consecration to the Divine; for when you can no more call anything, not even yourself, yours, when everything, including your body, sensations, feelings and thoughts belong to the Divine, the Divine takes the entire responsibility of all and you have nothing more to worry about.

WORK

If you want to be a true doer of divine works, your first aim must be to be totally free from all desire and self-regarding ego. All stress of egoistic choice, all hankering after personal profit, all stipulation of self-regarding desire must be extirpated from the nature. There must be no demand for fruit and no seeking for reward; the only fruit for you is the pleasure of the Divine Mother and the fulfilment of her work, your only reward a constant progression in divine consciousness and calm and strength and bliss.

*

To keep up work helps to keep the balance between the internal experience and the external development; otherwise one-sidedness and want of measure and balance may develop. Moreover, it is necessary to keep the sadhana of work for the Divine, because in the end that enables the sadhak to bring out the inner progress into the external nature and life and helps the integrality of the sadhana.

To go entirely inside in order to have experiences and to neglect the work, the external consciousness is to be unbalanced; so also to throw oneself outward and live in the external being alone is to be unbalanced. One must have the same consciousness in inner experience and outward action and make both full of the Mother.

There should be not only a general attitude, but each work should be offered to the Mother so as to keep the attitude a living one all the time.

*

The only work that spiritually purifies is that which is done without personal motives, without desire for fame or public recognition or worldly greatness, without insistence on one's own mental motives or vital lusts and demands or physical preferences, without vanity or crude self-assertion or claim for position or prestige, done for the sake of the Divine alone and at the command of the Divine.

*

Those who do work for the Mother in all sincerity, are prepared by the work itself for the right consciousness even if they do not sit down for meditation or follow any particular practice of Yoga. It is not necessary to tell you how to meditate; whatever is needful will come of itself if in your work and at all times you are sincere and keep yourself open to the Mother.

There is no stage of the sadhana in which works are impossible. A complete cessation of work and entire withdrawal into oneself is seldom advisable; it may encourage a too one-sided and visionary condition in which one lives in a sort of midworld of purely subjective experiences without a firm hold on either external reality or on the highest Reality and without the right use of the subjective experience to create a firm link and then a unification between the highest Reality and the external realisation in life.

*

Work for the Mother done with the right concentration on her is as much a sadhana as meditation and inner experiences.

To do both meditation and work and dedicate both to the Mother is the best thing.

*

The Mother does not think that it is good to give up all work and only read and meditate. Work is part of the Yoga and it gives the best opportunity for calling down the Presence, the Light and the Power into the vital and its activity; it increases also the field and the opportunity of surrender.

It is not enough to remember that the work is the Mother's — and the results also. You must learn to feel the Mother's force behind you and to open to the inspiration and the guidance. Always to remember by an effort of the mind is too difficult; but if you get into the consciousness in which you feel always the Mother's force in you or supporting you, that is the true thing.

*

Yoga through work is the easiest and most effective way to enter into the stream of this sadhana.

*

Work is not only for work's sake, but as field of sadhana for getting rid of the lower personality and its reactions and acquiring a full surrender to the Divine. As for the work itself, it must be done according to the organisation arranged or sanctioned by the

Mother. You must always remember that it is her work and not personally yours.

*

To leave your work is not a solution — it is through work that one can detect and progressively get rid of the feelings and movements that are contrary to the Yogic ideal — those of the ego. The test is to do the work given by the Mother without abhiman or insistence or personal choice of prestige, — not getting hurt by anything that touches the pride, or personal preference.

*

It is a great and high ideal that is put before the sadhak through work and it is not possible to realise it suddenly, but to grow steadily into it is possible, if one keeps the aim always before one — to be a selfless and perfectly tempered instrument for the work of the Divine Mother.

*

In work it is to do what is best for the work, without regard to one's own prestige or convenience, not to regard the work as one's own but as the Mother's, to do it according to rule, discipline, impersonal arrangement, even if conditions are not favourable to do the best according to the conditions, etc., etc.

*

The greater the difficulties that rise in the work the more one can profit by them in deepening the equality, if one takes it in the right spirit. You must also keep yourself open to receive the help towards that, for the help will always be coming from the Mother for the change of the nature.

*

If, however, the mind and the vital get the habit of opening to the Mother's Force, they are then supported by the Force and may even be fully filled with it — the Force does the work and the body feels no strain or fatigue before or after. But even then, unless the body itself is open and can absorb and keep the Force, sufficient rest in between the work is absolutely necessary. Otherwise, although the body may go on for a very long time, yet in the end there can be a danger of a collapse.

A complete freedom from fatigue is possible, but that comes only when there is a complete transformation of the law of the body by the full descent of a supramental Force into the earth-nature.

*

To work in the calm ever-widening consciousness is at once a sadhana and a siddhi.

*

The including of the outer consciousness in the transformation is of supreme importance in this Yoga — meditation cannot do it. Meditation can deal only with the inner being. So work is of primary importance — only it must be done with the right attitude and in the right consciousness, then it is as fruitful as any meditation can be.

*

The ignorance underlying this attitude is in the assumption that one must necessarily do only work or only meditation. Work by itself is only a preparation, so is meditation by itself, but work done in the increasing Yogic consciousness is a means of realisation as much as meditation is.

*

I have always said that work done as sadhana — done, that is to say, as an outflow of energy from the Divine and offered to the Divine or work done for the sake of the Divine or work done in a spirit of devotion is a powerful means of sadhana and that such work is especially necessary in this Yoga. By work and bhakti one can develop a consciousness in which eventually a natural meditation and realisation becomes possible.

*

All work done for the Divine is equally divine, manual labour done for the Divine is more divine than mental culture done for one's own development, fame or mental satisfaction. The idea of giving up physical work for mental self-development is a creation of the mental ego.

*

To be free from all egoistic motive, careful of truth in speech and action, void of self-will and self-assertion, watchful in all things, is the condition for being a flawless servant.

*

The work here is not intended for showing one's capacity or having a position or as a means of physical nearness to the Mother, but as a field and an opportunity for the Karmayoga — part of the integral Yoga, for learning to work in the true Yogic way, dedication through service, practical selflessness, obedience, scrupulousness, discipline, setting the Divine and the Divine's work first and oneself last, harmony, patience, forbearance, etc. When the workers learn these things and cease to be egocentric, as most of you are, then will come the time for work in which capacity can really be shown, although even then the showing of capacity will be an incident and can never be the main consideration or the object of divine work.

*

If too much work is done the quality of the work deteriorates in spite of the zest of the worker.

*

Mother does not disapprove of your writing a book — what she does not like is your being so lost in it that you can do nothing else. You must be master of what you do and not possessed by it.

*

You must do the work as an offering to the Divine and take it as part of your sadhana. In that spirit the nature of the work is of little importance and you can do any work without losing the contact with the inner presence.

All work done for the Divine, from poetry and art and music to carpentry or baking or sweeping a room, should be made perfect even in its smallest external detail as well as in the spirit in which it is done; for only then is it an altogether fit offering.

*

The truth is that you must not be subject to the ego or the external nature in your work. If you are, the work cannot form a part of the sadhana; instead, it becomes equivalent to trivial and ordinary work. Even the work must be done from within in a spirit of surrender.

The Mother:

To work for the Divine is to pray with the body.

*

Work done in the true spirit is meditation.

*

A good material work not exceeding normal capacities is most useful for keeping a good physical and moral poise.

*

Here, for each work given, the full strength and Grace are always given at the same time to do the work as it has to be done. If you do not feel the strength and the Grace it proves that there is some mistake in your attitude. The faith is lacking or you have fallen back on old tracks and old creeds and thus you lose all receptivity.

*

You will become more and more perfect in your work as the consciousness grows, increases, widens and is enlarged.

*

When in your work you find something giving trouble outside, look within and you will find in yourself the corresponding difficulty. Change yourself and the circumstances will change.

*

It is not so easy to do work. Don't think that somehow finishing the outward form of the work is doing the work in the true sense. It is much more difficult to work than to do "sadhana" as it is ordinarily understood. In meditation your consciousness goes higher and remains there in conditions of light and peace. In true work you have to do that also and much more. You have to do all that a Yogi does, you have to reach the highest heights and bring down those conditions of consciousness, light and peace and manifest them in your everyday jobs. For you no work is insignificant or trivial.

*

There must be order and harmony in your work. Mahasaraswati is not at all satisfied with your work if even the slightest disharmony, disorder or confusion are found in it. Even what is apparently the most insignificant thing must be done with perfect perfection, with a sense of cleanliness, beauty, harmony and order. For example even when you sweep a room you must try to make it as clean as a first class operation theatre.

*

Unless you work hard you do not get energy; because in that case you do not need it and don't deserve it. You get energy only when you make use of it.

OBSTACLES IN SADHANA

Attachment

If you are to do this Yoga, you must have only one desire and aspiration; you should make the submission and surrender sincere, real and complete. It cannot be as long as you cherish vital attachment to family, child or anything or anybody else.

*

In Yoga friendship can remain but attachment has to fall away or any such engrossing affection as would keep one tied to the ordinary life and consciousness.

*

Any attachment or restlessness comes in the way of a spiritual working. Train yourself to look calmly without disturbance and simply see what has to be done and quietly will it; it is so that the ordinary consent of the Nature-forces can be overtopped and overcome.

*

Even after the liberation, one has to remain vigilant for often these things go out and remain at a far distance, waiting to see if under any circumstances in any condition they can make a rush and recover their kingdom. If there has been an entire purification down to the depths and nothing is there to open the gate, then they cannot do it.

*

Attachment is attachment in whatever part of the being it may be. In order to be unattached one must be unattached everywhere, in the mental, vital and physical action.

*

To become indifferent to the attraction of outer objects is one of the first rules of Yoga, for this non-attachment liberates the inner being into peace and the true consciousness.

The Mother:

The attitude of the ascetic who says, "I want nothing" and the attitude of the man of the world who says, "I want this thing" are the same. The one may be as much attached to his renunciation as the other to his possession. You must accept all things — and only those things — that come from the Divine. Because things can come from concealed desires under disguise.

Desire

If desire is not mastered, how can there be any straight walking on the straight path? All desires and attachments are vital, all self-indulgence also. To reach the freedom without the discipline and development is given to few.

*

Ambition and vanity are things so natural to the human consciousness — they have even their use in ordinary life. But they have to be pushed out before one is far on this path — otherwise they are very dangerous attendants and can pervert both aspiration and siddhi.

*

If you entertain a desire, become impatient for the fruits of sadhana, then how will you remain peaceful and silent? A great work like the transformation of human nature, can it be done in a moment? Remain quiet, let the force of the Mother work in you, then in time everything will be accomplished.

The Mother:

First of all he must give up his desires whoever wants to follow this path; for desire is the most obscure and the most obscuring movement of the lower nature. Desires are motions of weakness and ignorance and they keep you chained to your weakness and to your ignorance. It is the same with all the lower impulses, jealousy or envy, hatred or violence, because they do not belong to the true nature of the Divine.

*

To conquer a desire brings more joy than to satisfy it.

*

Greed for anything concerning physical conveniences so-called necessities and comfort of whatever nature these are — is one of the most serious obstacles to sadhana. Each little satisfaction you get through greed is one step backward from the goal.

Despondency

Depression prevents the Force from flowing through and calls in the adverse forces and gives them a chance to destroy the helpful formations that are made. However or from wheresoever it came, the only thing to do with a depression is to throw it out.

These feelings of despair and exaggerated sense of self-depreciation and helplessness are suggestions of a hostile Force and should never be admitted. The transformation of the external being is the most difficult part of the Yoga and it demands faith, patience, quietude and firm determination.

One must be more obstinate than the obstinate material nature and persevere until the light and truth can take permanent hold of the parts which are still responsive to the old movements.

*

The sadder you are and the more you lament, the farther you go away from me. The Divine is not sad and for realising the Divine you must reject far from yourself all sadness and all sentimental weakness.

*

A depression is always unreasonable and it leads nowhere. It is the most subtle enemy of the Yoga.

Be courageous and do not think so much of yourself. It is because you make your little ego the centre of your preoccupation that you are sad and unsatisfied. To forget oneself is the great remedy for all ills.

Difficulties, Disturbances

Do not be troubled by your surroundings and their oppositions.

These conditions are often imposed at first as a kind of ordeal. If you can remain tranquil and undisturbed and continue your sadhana without allowing yourself to be inwardly troubled under these circumstances, it will help to give you a much needed strength; for the path of Yoga is always beset with inner and outer difficulties and the sadhaka must develop a quiet, firm and solid strength to meet them.

*

All who enter the spiritual path have to face the difficulties and ordeals of the path, those which rise from their own nature and those which come in from outside. The difficulties in the nature always rise again and again till you overcome them; they must be faced with both strength and patience. But the vital part is prone to depression when ordeals and difficulties rise. But you must train yourself to overcome this reaction of depression, calling in the Mother's Force to aid you.

All who cleave to the path steadfastly can be sure of their spiritual destiny. If anyone fails to reach it, it can only be for one of the two reasons, either because they leave the path or because for some lure of ambition, vanity, desire, etc. they go astray from the sincere dependence on the Divine.

*

The Divine is there, but He does not ignore the conditions, the laws, the circumstances of Nature; it is under these conditions that He does all His work, His work in the world and in man and consequently also in the sadhaka, the aspirant, even in the God-knower and God-lover; even the saint and the sage continue to have difficulties and to be limited by their human nature.

*

In the ordinary life people accept the vital movements, anger, desire, greed, sex, etc. as natural, allowable and legitimate things, part of the human nature. Only so far as society discourages them or insists to keep them within fixed limits or subject to a decent restraint or measure, people try to control them so as to conform to the social standard of morality or rule of conduct. Here, on the contrary, as in all spiritual life, the conquest and complete mastery of these things is demanded. That is why the struggle is more felt, not because these things rise more strongly in sadhaks than in ordinary men, but because of the intensity of the struggle between the spiritual mind which demands control and the vital movements which rebel and want to continue in the new as they did in the old life.

*

You should know perfectly well that, in our Yoga, pain and suffering and struggle and excesses of despair are natural — though not inevitable on the way — not because they are helps but because they are imposed on us by the darkness of this human nature out of which we have to struggle into the Light.

*

Nobody has ever said that the spiritual change was an easy thing; all spiritual seekers will say that it is difficult but supremely worth doing. If one's desire for the Divine has become the master desire, then surely one can give one's whole life to it without repining and not grudge the time, difficulty or labour.

*

That does not mean that those whose faith is not so strong or surrender complete cannot arrive, but usually they have at first to go by small steps and to face the difficulties of their nature until by perseverance or tapasya they make a sufficient opening. Even a faltering faith and a slow and partial surrender have their force and their result, otherwise only the rare few could do sadhana at all.

*

Obstacles are there — they are part of Nature and they have to be overcome. The Mother's help is always there but you are not conscious of it except when the psychic is active and the consciousness not clouded.

*

He is quite right in saying that the heaviness of these attacks was due to the fact that you had taken up the sadhana in earnest and were approaching, as one might say, the gates of the Kingdom of Light. That always makes these forces rage and they strain every nerve and use or create every opportunity to turn the sadhak back or, if possible, drive him out of the path altogether by their suggestions, their violent influences and their exploitations of all kinds of incidents that always crop up more and more when these conditions prevail, so that he may not reach the gates.... People nowadays seek the explanation for everything in their ignorant reason, their surface experience and in outside happenings. They do not see the hidden forces and inner causes.... These forces find their *point d'appui* in the sadhak himself, in the ignorant parts of his consciousness and its assent to their suggestions and influences....

*

It is inevitable once one enters into this Yoga that the difficulties should rise up and they go on rising up so long as anything of them is left in the system at all. What is needed to pass through difficulties is sincerity and perseverance.

*

This Yoga is a spiritual battle; its very attempt raises all sorts of adverse forces and one must be ready to face difficulties, sufferings, reverses of all sorts in a calm unflinching spirit.

*

The difficulties that come are ordeals and tests and if one meets them in the right spirit, one comes out stronger and spiritually purer and greater.

*

When there is an attack from the human instruments of adverse forces, one should try to overcome it not in a spirit of personal hatred or anger or wounded egoism, but with a calm spirit of strength and equanimity and a call to the Divine Force to act. Success or failure lies with the Divine.

One should then seek out this weakness in oneself and correct it. No weakness, no arrogance or violence, this should be the spirit.

*

When difficulties arise, remain quiet within and call down the Mother's Force to remove them. The Mother's Force is not only above on the summit of the being. It is there with you and near you, ready to act whenever your nature will allow it. It is so with everybody here.

*

However strong the attack may be, and even if it overcomes for the time being, still it will rapidly pass away if you have formed the habit of opening to the Mother. The peace will come back if you remain quiet and keep yourself open to it and to the Force. Once something of the Truth has shown itself within you, it will always, even if for a time heavily clouded over with wrong movements, shine out again like the sun in heaven. Therefore persevere with confidence and never lose courage.

*

Outer difficulties or inconveniences you should not allow to alarm or depress you. Inner difficulties should also be met with detachment, calm, equality, the unshakable will to conquer. These small desires obstruct greatly the change in the outer consciousness and the being must be free from them if the transformation is not to be hampered there.

*

A solid mind, a solid nervous system, and a steady psychic flame seem to be the only safeguard against "terrible attacks" in sadhana. If such things did not happen there would be no need of a fight day and night.

*

It is a period when doubt, denial, dryness, greyness and all kindred things come up with a great force and often reign completely for a time. It is after this stage has been successfully crossed that the true light begins to come, the light which is not of the mind but of the spirit. It does not really indicate any radical disability in the nature but certainly it is a hard ordeal and one has to stick very firmly to pass through it.

*

This always comes in the way when one wants to progress in one's sadhana, but in the end if one is sincere in one's aspiration these troubles help to prepare the victory of the soul over all that opposes.

*

The real difficulty is always in ourselves, not in our surroundings. There are three things necessary in order to make men invincible: Will, Disinterestedness and Faith. We may have a will to emancipate ourselves, but sufficient faith may be lacking. We may have faith in our ultimate emancipation, but the will to use the necessary means may be wanting. And even if there are will and faith, we may use them with a violent attachment to the fruit of our work or with passions of hatred, blind excitement or hasty forcefulness which may produce evil reactions. For this reason it is necessary, in a work of such magnitude, to have resort to a higher Power than that of mind and body in order to overcome unprecedented obstacles. This is the need of Sadhana.

*

The path is long, but self-surrender makes it short; the way is difficult, but perfect trust makes it easy. The force that can do it, exists. But it is hidden in a secret chamber within us and of that chamber God holds the key. Let us find Him and claim it.

The Mother:

The difficulties are always due to a resistance, some part or several parts of the being refusing to receive the force, the consciousness and the light put upon them and revolting against the divine influence. But to keep steady one's aspiration and to look at oneself with an absolute sincerity are the sure means to overcome all obstacles.

*

When you feel unhappy like that, it means that you have a progress to make. You can say that we always need to progress; it is true. But at times our nature gives its consent to the needed change and then everything goes smoothly, even happily. On the contrary, sometimes the part that has to progress refuses to move and clings to its old habits through ignorance, inertia, attachment or desire. Then, under the pressure of the perfecting Force, the struggle starts translating itself into unhappiness or revolt, or both together.

The only remedy is to keep quiet, look within oneself honestly to find out what is wrong and set to work courageously to put it right; and the more sincere your endeavour, the more the Divine consciousness will help and assist you.

*

Don't let anything from outside approach and disturb you. What people think, do or say is of little importance. The only thing that counts is your relation with the Divine.

*

The sufferings and miseries are not meant for the benefit of their souls, it is only very strong beings who can find an inner benefit in sufferings; they are the result of the world's resistance to the Divine action. The best each sadhak can do is to conquer in himself this resistance.

Ego, Vanity, Pride

Efface the stamp of ego from the heart and let the love of the Mother take its place. Cast from the mind all insistence on your personal ideas and judgment, then you will have the wisdom to understand her. Let there be no obsession of self-will, ego-drive in the action, love of personal authority, attachment to personal preference, then the Mother's force will be able to act clearly in you and you will get the inexhaustible energy for which you ask and your service will be perfect.

*

The sooner you get rid of abhiman the better. Anyone who

indulges abhiman (ego) puts himself under the influence of the hostile forces.

*

Pride is only one form of ego — there are then ten thousand others. Every action of man is full of ego — the good ones as well as the bad, his humility as much as his pride, his virtues as much as his vices.

To get the ego out of the human nature is not so simple as that. If one is free from ego, does nothing with reference to himself or for his own sake but only for the Divine and all his thoughts and feelings are for the Divine, then he is Jivanmukta and a Siddha Yogi.

*

The egoism of the instrument can be as dangerous or more dangerous to spiritual progress than the egoism of the doer. The ego-sense is contrary to spiritual realisation. There should be no big I, not even a small one.

*

For the ego, however insistent it may be, one has to keep one's eye on it and say no to all its suggestions so that each position it takes up proves to be a fruitless move. It is only by a constant quiet vigilance and increasing consciousness that it can be got out — for if it is not allowed to play, it conceals itself and takes subtle and disguised forms.

*

Without the liberation of the psychic and the realisation of the true Self the ego cannot go, both are necessary. Liberation comes by loss of ego and desire. To get rid of ego is as difficult as to make complete surrender.

*

Very few people in the Ashram are conscious of their ego-centricity. They are all ego-centric and they do not realise their ego-centricity. Even in their sadhana the 'I' is always there, — my sadhana, my progress, my everything. The remedy is to think constantly of the Divine, not of oneself, to work, to act, do sadhana for the Divine; not to consider how this or that affects me personally, not to claim anything, but to refer all to the Divine.

*

The ego-centric man feels and takes things as they affect him. Does this please me or displease, give me gladness or pain, flatter my pride, vanity, ambition or hurt it, satisfy my desires or thwart them, etc. The unegoistic man does not look at things like that. He looks to see what things are in themselves and would be if he were not there, what is their meaning, how they fit into the scheme of things — or else he feels calm and equal, refers everything to the Divine. There can be many points of view which are not ego-centric.

*

Self-justification keeps the wrong movement going because it gives a mental support. Self-justification is always a sign of ego and ignorance. When one has a wider consciousness, one knows that each one has his own way of looking at things and finds in that way his own justification, so that both parties in a quarrel believe themselves to be in the right. It is only when one looks from above in a consciousness clear of ego that one sees all sides of a thing and also their real truth.

*

It is the petty ego in each that likes to discover and talk about the "real or unreal" defects of others. The ego has no right to judge them, because it has not the right view or the right spirit. It is only the calm, disinterested, dispassionate, all-compassionate and all-loving Spirit that can judge and see rightly the strength and weakness in each being.

*

When a dangerous habit of constant self-justification becomes strong in the sadhak, it is impossible to turn him in this part of his being to the right consciousness and action because at each step his whole preoccupation is to justify himself. His mind rushes at once to maintain his own idea, his own position or his own course of action. This he is ready to do by any kind of argument, sometimes the most clumsy and foolish.

*

This Yoga can only be done to the end by those who are in total earnest about it and ready to abolish their little human ego and its demands in order to find themselves in the Divine. It cannot be done in a spirit of levity or laxity; the work is too high and difficult, the adverse powers in the lower Nature too ready to take advantage of the least sanction or the smallest opening, the aspiration and tapasya needed too constant and intense.

*

All ambition, pride and vanity must disappear from the thoughts and the feelings. All falsehood must be rejected from the speech, thought and action and all ostentation, arrogance and insolence.

*

The earth-consciousness does not want to change so it rejects what comes down to it from above — it has always done so. It is only if those who have taken this Yoga open themselves and are willing to change their lower nature that this unwillingness can disappear.

*

What stands in the way of course is always the vital ego with its ignorance and the pride of its ignorance and the physical consciousness with its inertia which resents and resists any call to change and its indolence which does not like to take the trouble — it finds it more comfortable to go on its own way repeating always the same old movements and, at best, expecting everything to be done for it in some way or at some time.

*

The first thing is to have the right inner attitude; the rest is the will to transform oneself and the vigilance to perceive and reject all that belongs to the ego and the tamasic persistence of the lower nature. Finally, to keep oneself always open to the Mother in every part of the being so that the process of transformation may find no hindrance.

*

Egoism is part of the machinery — a tool of the universal forces. It is only when one gets into touch with a higher Nature that it is possible to get free of this rule of ego and subjection to these forces.

*

The ego is by its nature a smallness of being; it brings contraction of the consciousness and with the contraction limitation of knowledge, disabling ignorance, — confinement and a diminution of power and by that diminution incapacity and weakness — scission of oneness and by that scission disharmony and failure of sympathy and love and understanding, — inhibition or fragmentation of delight of being and by that fragmentation pain and sorrow. To recover what is lost we must break out of the worlds of ego.

The Mother:

Those who are capable of extending the consciousness as wide as the world, become the world; but those who are shut up in their little bodies and limited feelings stop at those limits; their bodies and their petty feelings are to them their whole self.

*

If you are truly surrendered to the Divine, in the right manner and totally, then at every moment you will be what you ought to be, you will do what you ought to do, you will know what you ought to know. But for that you should have transcended all the limitations of ego.

*

To feel hurt by what others do or think or say is always a sign of weakness and proof that the whole being is not exclusively turned towards the Divine, not under the divine influence alone. And then instead of bringing with oneself the divine atmosphere made of love, tolerance, understanding, patience, it is one's ego that throws itself in response to another's with stiffness and hurt feelings and the disharmony is aggravated.

Fear

All dread of fire or other violent forces should be overcome. For dread shows a weakness — the free spirit can stand fearless before even the biggest forces of Nature.

*

If you are afraid of the hostile forces when they try to come, you expose yourself to their power.

The Mother:

Once you enter the path of Yoga you must get rid of all fears — the fears of your mind, the fears of your vital, the fears of your body which are lodged in its very cells. One who seeks the transformation and is a follower of the Path, must become through and through fearless, not to be touched or shaken by anything whatever in any part of his nature.

*

Generally speaking, the greatest obstacle perhaps that hinders man's progress is fear. Of all kinds of fear the most subtle and the most clinging is that of death. One can conquer that alone which one fears not, and he who fears death has already been vanquished by Death.

The first and the most important thing is to know that life is one and immortal. Only the forms, countless in number, are transient and brittle. Life then does not die; but the forms are dissolved, and it is this dissolution that the physical consciousness fears. And yet the form changes constantly and there is nothing that debars this change from being progressive.

One who craves for death may have to wait long to get it and one who fears it may be struck down suddenly in spite of all precautions taken....

*

Beyond all the emotions, in the silent and quiet depths of our being, there is a light burning constantly, the light of the psychic consciousness. Go in search of this light, concentrate upon it; it is with you . With a persevering will you will surely find it. As soon as you enter into it, you awake to the sense of immortality. You feel you have always lived, you will live always.

Food

It is the attachment to food, the greed and eagerness for it, making it an unduly important thing in the life, that is contrary to the spirit of Yoga. To be aware that something is pleasant to the palate is not wrong; only one must have no desire nor hankering for it. There should be neither eagerness nor repugnance. To be always thinking about food and troubling the mind is quite the wrong way of getting rid of the food-desire.

*

Do not trouble your mind about food. Take it in the right quantity (neither too much nor too little), without greed or repulsion, as the means given you by the Mother for the maintenance of the body, in the right spirit, offering it to the Divine in you.

*

It is no part of this Yoga to suppress taste, rasa, altogether. What is to be got rid of is vital desire and attachment, the greed of food, being overjoyed at getting the food you like, sorry and discontented when you do not have it, giving an undue importance to it. Equality is here the test as in so many other matters.

*

It is not necessary to have desire or greed of food in order to eat. The Yogi eats not out of desire, but to maintain the body. It is a mistake to neglect the body and let it waste away; the body is the means of the sadhana and should be maintained in good order. There should be no attachment to it, but no contempt or neglect either of the material part of our nature.

*

Spiritually, I should say that the effect of food depends more on the occult atmosphere and influences that come with it than on anything in the food itself. Vegetarianism is another question altogether; it stands, on a will not to do harm to the more conscious forms of life for the satisfaction of the belly.

*

No Yoga can be done without sufficient food and sleep. Fasting or sleeplessness makes the nerves morbid and excited and weaken the brain and lead to delusions and fantasies.

Fasting is not permissible in the Ashram, as its practice is more often harmful than helpful to the spiritual endeavour.

*

Prolonged fasting may lead to an excitation of the nervous being which often brings vivid imaginations and hallucinations that are taken for true experiences; such fasting is frequently suggested by the vital Entities, because it puts the consciousness into an unbalanced state which favours their designs. It is therefore discouraged here.

*

Too much eating makes the body material and heavy, eating too little makes it weak and nervous — one has to find the true harmony and balance between the body's need and the food taken.

The Mother:

It is an inner attitude of freedom from attachment and from greed of food and desire of the palate that is needed, not undue diminution of the quantity taken or any self-starvation. One must take sufficient food for the maintenance of the body and its strength and health but without attachment or desire.

*

That is what happens along with the meal that you take, you absorb also, in a large or small measure, the consciousness of the animal whose flesh you swallow. Of course it is nothing serious, but it is not always pleasant. Yet obviously it does not help you to be more on the side of man than on that of the animal kind. Primitive men, we know, were much nearer the animal level and used to take raw meat: that gave them evidently more strength and energy than cooked meat.... Also it was for this reason perhaps that there was in their intestines an organ called the appendix in a much bigger size than it is now: for it had to digest raw meat. As men, however, started cooking their food and found it more tasty that way, the organ too gradually diminished in size and fell into atrophy; now it does not serve any purpose, it is an encumbrance and often a source of illness. This means that it is time to change the diet and take to something less bestial. It depends, however, on the state of the consciousness of each person. An ordinary man, who leads an ordinary life, has ordinary aspirations, thinks of nothing else than earning his livelihood, keeping good health and rearing a family, need not pick and choose, except on purely hygienic grounds. He may eat meat or anything else that he considers helpful and useful, doing good to him.

But if you wish to move from the ordinary life to a higher life, the problem acquires an interest. And again, for a higher life if you wish to move up still farther and prepare yourself for transformation, then the problem becomes very important. For there are certain foods that help the body to become more refined and others that keep it down to the level of animalhood. But it is only then that the question acquires an importance, not before. Before you come to that point, you have a lot of other things to do. It is certainly better to purify your mind, purify your vital before you think of purifying your body....

You must begin from within. I have said a hundred times, you must begin from above. You must purify first the higher region and then purify the lower. I do not mean by this that you should give yourself up to all the licences that degrade the body. I am not advising you not to control your desires. What I mean is this: do not try to be an angel in the body before you are already something of the kind in your mind and in your vital. For that will bring about a dislocation, a lack of balance.

Hostile Forces

The hostile forces make it their function to attack and disturb the sadhaks, but if there were no wrong movement and no imperfection and weakness, they should not be disturbed.

*

Tests are applied not by the Divine but by the forces of the lower planes — mental, vital, physical — and allowed by the Divine because that is part of the soul's training and helps it to know itself, its powers and limitations it has to outgrow. The Mother is not testing you at every moment, but rather helping you at every moment to rise beyond the necessity of tests and difficulties which belong to the inferior consciousness.

*

Those who fall, fall not because of the attacks of the vital forces, but because they put themselves on the side of the hostile Forces and prefer a vital ambition or desire to the spiritual siddhi.

*

Hostile forces attack every sadhak; some are conscious of it, others are not. Their object is either to influence the person or to use him or to spoil his sadhana or the work or any other motive of the kind. Their object is not to test, but their attack may be used by the guiding power as a test.

*

The hostile forces do not need a cause for attacking — they attack whenever and whoever they can. What one has to see is that nothing responds or admits them.

*

There are no sadhaks who are never attacked by wrong forces — but if one has a complete faith and self-consecration, one can throw off the attack without too much difficulty.

*

The hostile forces are there in the world to maintain the Ignorance — they were there in the sadhana, because they had the right to test the sincerity of the sadhaks in their power and will to cleave to the Divine and overcome all difficulties. But this is only so long as the higher Light has not descended into the physical.

*

In Yoga, as in every great or serious human effort, there is always bound to be an abundance of adverse interventions and unfavourable circumstances which have to be overcome. To give them too great an importance increases their importance and their power to multiply themselves, gives them, as it were, confidence in themselves and the habit of coming. To face them with equanimity, diminishes their importance and effect and in the end, though not at once, gets rid of their persistence and recurrence. It is therefore a principle in Yoga to recognise the determining power of what is within us — for that is the deeper truth — to set that right and establish the inward strength as against the power of outward circumstances. The strength is there — even in the weakest; one has to find it, to unveil it and to keep it in front throughout the journey and the battle.

*

About the attacks and the action of the cosmic forces — these attacks very ordinarily become violent when the progress is becoming rapid and on the way to be definite — specially if they find they cannot carry out an effective aggression into the inner being, they try to shake by outside assault. One must take it as a trial of strength, a call for gathering all one's capacities of calm and openness to the Light and Power, so as to make oneself an instrument for the victory of the Divine over the undivine, of the Light over the darkness in the world tangle. It is in this spirit that you must face these difficulties till the higher things are so confirmed in you that these forces can attack no longer.

*

In the cosmos, there are the higher forces of the Divine Nature — the forces of Light, Truth, divine Power, Peace, Ananda — there are the forces of the lower nature which belong either to a lower truth or to ignorance and error — there are also the hostile forces whose whole aim is to maintain the reign of Darkness, Falsehood, Death and Suffering as the law of life.

The Mother:

Attacks from adverse forces are inevitable: you have to take them as tests on your way and go courageously through the ordeal. The struggle may be hard, but when you come out of it, you have gained something, you have advanced a step. There is even a necessity for the existence of the hostile forces. They make your determination stronger, your aspiration clearer.

*

If the attack takes the form of adverse suggestions try quietly to push them away, as you would some material object. The quieter you are, the stronger you become. The firm basis of all spiritual power is equanimity. You must not allow anything to disturb your poise: you can then resist every attack.

The only way to fail in your battle with the hostile forces is not to have a true confidence in the Divine help. Sincerity in the aspiration always brings down the required succour.

Human Nature or Prakriti

Most men are, like animals, driven by the forces of Nature: whatever desires come, they fulfil them, whatever emotions come they allow them to play, whatever physical wants they have, they try to satisfy. We say then that the activities and feelings of men are controlled by their Prakriti, and mostly by the vital and physical nature. The body is the instrument of the Prakriti or Nature — it obeys its own nature or it obeys the vital forces of desires, passion etc.

But man has also a mind and, as he develops, he learns to control his vital and physical nature by his reason and by his will. This control is very partial: for the reason is often deluded by vital desires and the ignorance of the physical and it puts itself on their side and tries to justify by its ideas, reasonings or arguments their mistakes and wrong movements. Even if the reason keeps free and tells the vital or the body, "Do not do this," yet the vital and the body often follow their own movement in spite of the prohibition — man's mental will is not strong enough to compel them.

*

When people do sadhana, there is a higher Nature that works within, the psychic and spiritual, and they have to put their nature under the influence of the psychic being and the higher spiritual self or of the Divine. Not only the vital and the body but the mind also has to learn the Divine Truth and obey the divine rule.

But because of the lower nature and its continued hold on them, they are unable at first and for a long time to prevent their nature from following the old ways — even when they know or are told from within what to do or what not to do. It is only by persistent sadhana, by getting into the higher spiritual consciousness and spiritual nature that this difficulty can be overcome; but even for the strongest and best sadhaks it takes a long time.

*

The lower nature is ignorant and undivine, not in itself hostile but shut to the Light and Truth. The hostile forces are anti-divine, not merely undivine; they make use of the lower nature, pervert it, fill it with distorted movements and by that means influence man and even try to enter and possess or at least entirely control him.

*

The rule in Yoga is not to let the depression depress you, to stand back from it, observe its cause and remove the cause. The Yogi should look on all the defects of the nature as movements of the lower prakriti common to all and reject them calmly, firmly and persistently with full confidence in the Divine Power. However hard the fight, the only thing is to fight it out now and here to the end.

*

The Mother does not make people commit mistakes; it is the Prakriti that makes them do it — if the Purusha does not refuse his consent. The Mother here is not this lower Prakriti, but the Divine Shakti and it is her work to press on this lower Nature to change. You can say that under the pressure, the Prakriti stumbles and is unable to reply perfectly and makes mistakes. But it is not the Mother who makes you do wrong movements or does the wrong movements in you.

Everything comes from the Divine; but the lower Prakriti is the power of the ignorance — it is not therefore a power of truth, but only of mixed truth and falsehood. The Mother here stands not for the Power of Ignorance, but for the Power that has come down to bring down the Truth and raise up to the Truth out of the Ignorance.

*

The Cosmic Force is a Power that works under the conditions of the Ignorance — it appears as the lower nature and the lower nature makes you do wrong things. The Divine allows the play of these forces so long as you do not yourself want anything better. But if you are a sadhak, then you do not accept the play of the lower nature, you turn to the Divine Mother instead, and ask her to work through you instead of the lower nature. It is only when you have turned entirely in every part of your being to the Divine Mother and to her alone that the Divine will do all actions through you.

*

The character is made up of habits and it clings to them, is disposed to think them the very law of its being and it is a hard job to get it to change at all except under a strong pressure of circumstances. Especially in the physical parts, the body, the physical mind, the physical life movements, there is this resistance; the tamasic element in Nature is powerful there, what the Gita describes as *aprakāśa*, absence of light, and *apravṛtti*, a tendency to inertia, inactivity, unwillingness to make an effort and, as a result, even when the effort is made, a constant readiness to doubt, to despond and despair, to give up, renounce the aim and the endeavour, collapse.

*

Physical consciousness wants the satisfaction of the ego, "self-fulfilment", appreciation, the granting of its desires. It measures the Divine Love by the outward favours showered upon it and looks jealously to see who gets more of these favours than itself, then says that the Divine has no love for it and assigns reasons which are either derogatory to the Divine, or self-depreciation and cause for despair. It is tamasic and does not want to change, does not want to believe unless it can be done by reassuring the vital ego; it is part of human nature and has always been there, hampering and limiting the sadhana. Its existence is no reason for despair — everyone has it and the sadhana has to be done in spite of it, in spite of the mixture it brings till the time comes when it has to be definitely rejected. It is difficult to do it, but perfectly possible.

*

Human nature is shot through in all its stuff with the thread of the ego; even when one tries to get away from it, it is in front or could be behind all the thoughts and actions like a shadow. To see that is the first step, to discern the falsity and absurdity of the ego-movements is the second, to discourage and refuse it at each step is the third, — but it goes entirely only when one sees, experiences and lives the One in everything and equally everywhere.

*

One must not treat the human nature like a machine to be handled according to rigid mental rules — a great plasticity is needed in dealing with its complex motives.

The sadhana is done by the Mother according to the Truth and necessity of each nature and of each plane of Nature.

*

It was inevitable that in the course of the sadhana these inferior parts of the nature should be brought forward in order that like the rest of the being they may make the crucial choice and either accept or refuse transformation. My whole work depends upon this movement; it is the decisive ordeal of this Yoga. If the little external personality is to persist in retaining its obscure and limited, its petty and ignoble, its selfish and false and stupid human consciousness, this amounts to a flat negation of the work and the sadhana.

*

I suppose if the Nirvana aim had been put before the disciples, more would have been fit for it, for the Nirvana aim is easier than the one we have put before us — and they would not have found it so difficult to reach the standard. The sadhaks here are of all kinds and in all stages. But the real difficulty even for those who have progressed is with the external man. Even among those who follow the old ideal, the external man of the sadhak remains almost the same even after they have attained to something. The inner being gets free, the outer follows still its fixed nature. Our Yoga can succeed only if the external man too changes, but that is the most difficult of all things. It is only by a change, of the physical nature that it can be done, by a descent of the higher light into this lower part of Nature. It is here that the struggle is going on. The internal being of most of the sadhaks here, however imperfect still, is still different from that of the ordinary man, but the external still clings to its old ways, manners, habits. It is when this is realised and done, that the Yoga will produce its full results in the Ashram itself, and not before.

*

People with small and narrow minds are in love with their narrowness and attached to their own limited ideas, feelings, opinions, preferences and get disturbed, angry or full of doubt if anyone tries to make them think more widely.

The Mother:

Among human beings, the most widely spread disease is mental narrowness. They understand only what is in their own consciousness and cannot tolerate anything else.

Mind

It is not possible to make a foundation in Yoga if the mind is restless. The first thing needed is quiet in the mind. Also to merge the personal consciousness is not the first aim of the Yoga; the first aim is to open it to a higher spiritual consciousness and for this also a quiet mind is the first need.

*

People do not understand what I write because the mind by itself cannot understand things that are beyond it. People often catch hold of something written by me or said by the Mother, give it an interpretation quite other than or far beyond its true meaning and deduce from it a suddenly extreme and logical conclusion which is quite contrary to our knowledge and experience.

*

In this Yoga one is supposed to go beyond every mental idealistic culture. Ideas and Ideals belong to the mind and are half-truths only; the mind too is, more often than not, satisfied with merely having an ideal, with the pleasure of idealising while life remains always the same, untransformed or changed only a little and mostly in appearance. The spiritual seeker does not turn aside from the pursuit of realisation to mere idealising; not to idealise, but to realise the Divine Truth is always his aim, either beyond or in life also — and in the latter case it is necessary to transform mind and life which cannot be done without surrender to the action of the Divine Force, the Mother.

*

The Divine Consciousness acts from a light that is beyond that level of human consciousness which makes the human standard of these things. It acts for and from a greater good than the apparent good men follow after. It acts also according to a greater truth than men conceive. It is for this reason that the human mind cannot understand the divine action and its motives — he must first rise into a higher consciousness and be in spiritual contact or union with the Divine.

*

The mind acts according to hard and fast rules and standards, while the spirit sees the truth of all and the truth of each and acts variously according to its own comprehensive and complex vision. That is why we say that no one can understand by his personal mental judgment the Mother's actions and reasons for action: it can only be understood by entering into the larger consciousness from which she sees things and acts upon them. That is baffling to the mind because it uses its small measures, but that is the truth of the matter.

*

The weak-willed man is governed by his vital and physical impulsions, his mental being is not dynamic enough to make its will prevail over them. His will is not "free" because it is not strong enough to be free, it is the slave of the forces that act on or in his vital and physical nature.

*

Thoughts, ideas, etc. are always wandering about, seeking a mind that may embody them. One mind takes, looks, rejects — another takes, looks, accepts. Two different minds catch the same thought-form or thought-wave, but the mental activities being different, make different results out of them, and the recipient cries proudly, "I, I have done this". Ego, Sir! ego! You are the recipient, the conditioning medium, if you like — but nothing more.

*

Nothing is more dangerous than the influences of the physical mind trying to build up conclusions upon outward appearances — they have nine chances out of ten of being false. One must learn to distrust hasty conclusions from surface appearances and learn to see and know things from within.

*

In ordinary life people always judge wrongly because they judge by mental standards and generally by conventional standards. The human mind is an instrument not of truth but of ignorance and error.

*

The insistence of the ordinary mind and its wrong reasonings, sentiments and judgments, the random activity of the thinking mind in concentration or its mechanical activity, the slowness of response to the veiled or the initial touch are the ordinary obstacles the mind imposes, just as pride, ambition, vanity, sex, greed, grasping of things for one's own ego are the difficulties and obstacles offered by the vital. As the vital difficulties can be fought down and conquered, so can the mental. Only one has to see that these are the inevitable obstacles and neither cling to them nor be terrified or overwhelmed because they are there. One has to persevere till one can stand back from the mind as from the vital.

*

A thousand questions can be asked about anything whatsoever, but to answer would require a volume, and even then the mind would understand nothing. It is only by a growth in the consciousness itself that you can get some direct perception of these things. But for that the mind must be quiet and a direct feeling and intuition take its place.

*

That trouble is from the physical mind refusing to take the trouble of the labour and struggle necessary for the spiritual achievement. It wants to get the highest, but desires a smooth course all the way, "who the devil is going to face so much trouble for getting the Divine?" — that is the underlying feeling. It is only when one has cleared the field and ploughed and sown and watched over it that big harvests can be hoped for.

*

All things are the Divine because the Divine is there, but hidden not manifest; when the mind goes out to things, it is not with the sense of the Divine in them, but for the appearances only which conceal the Divine. It is necessary therefore for you as a sadhak to turn entirely to the Mother in whom the Divine is manifest and not run after the appearances, the desire of which or the interest in which prevents you from meeting the Divine. Once the being is consecrated, then it can see the Divine everywhere — and then it can include all things in the one consciousness without a separate interest or desire.

*

To be rid of the external mind and its doubts one must cease to be attached to or accept its ideas in the feelings of the vital. One must realise that those things are ignorance, not knowledge, and that there is a true consciousness and true knowledge which come only by quietude of the mind and vital and one must aspire to that.

*

The thinking mind has to learn how to be entirely silent. It is only then that true knowledge can come.

The Mother:

The mind is not an instrument for knowledge. Its true role is to give a form, to initiate an action. It is mind that puts in order the different elements of the inspiration and organises the action....

Knowledge does not come from the mind. It comes from the profundities of the soul or from a higher consciousness. Man's role is to concentrate this knowledge in the physical world and organise it in order to give action a rational basis....

Mind has a powerful control over all vital impulses. Because of it, all that comes from the vital world can be used for a disciplined and organised action.

But for that, it must be at the service of some other thing, of a higher ideal, or of a divine consciousness and must not remain satisfied with itself.

These are the two roles of the mind. It is a force, an instrument for control. And when it is sufficiently developed it becomes a very powerful and capable instrument for organisation and for formation.

Relationship

Relations after taking up Yoga should be less and less based on a physical origin or the habits of the physical consciousness and more and more on the basis of sadhana. Family ties create an unnecessary interchange and come in the way of a complete turning to the Divine.

Child-parent relation is a law of human society, not a law of Karma. The child did not ask the father to bring him into the world and if the father has done it for his own pleasure, it is the least he can do to bring up the child. All these are social relations, but whatever they are, they cease once one takes to the spiritual life. It is the Divine alone with whom one has to do.

The Mother:

One who has given himself to the Divine has no longer any other duty than to make that consecration more and more perfect. The world and those who live in it have always wanted to put human — social and family — duty before duty to the Divine, which they have stigmatised as egoism. How indeed could they judge otherwise, they who have no experience of the reality of the Divine? But for the Divine regard their opinion has no value, their will has no force. These are movements of ignorance, nothing more. You should not attempt to convince; above all, you should not let yourself be touched or shaken. You must shut yourself carefully within your ivory tower of consecration and attend from the Divine alone help, protection, guidance and approbation. To be condemned by the whole world is nothing to him who knows that he has the approval of the Divine and his support.

*

All that is based on human relationship is unstable and transient, mixed and unsatisfactory; it is only what is established in the Divine and through the Divine that can last and give satisfaction.

Sex

The sadhaka has to turn away entirely from the invasion of the vital and the physical by the sex-impulse — for, if he does not conquer the sex-impulse there can be no settling in the body of the divine consciousness and the divine Ananda.

*

This Yoga demands a full ascension of the whole lower or ordinary consciousness to join the spiritual above it and a full descent of the spiritual into the mind, life and body to transform it. The total ascent is impossible so long as sex-desire blocks the way; the descent is dangerous so long as sex-desire is powerful in the vital. One must, therefore, clear this obstacle out of the way; otherwise there is either no safety or no free movement towards finality in the sadhana.

To eliminate it one must first be careful to harbour no sexual imagination or feeling in the waking state, next, to put a strong will on the body and especially on the sexual centre that there should be nothing of the kind in sleep.

*

Inactivity is an atmosphere in which sex easily rises.

*

There are a number of women who can love with the mind, the psychic, the vital (heart), but they shrink from a touch on the body and even when that goes, the physical act remains abhorrent to them. They may yield under pressure, but it does not reconcile them to the act which always seems to them animal and degrading. Women know this, but men seem to find it hard to believe; but it is perfectly true.

*

The one serious matter is the sex-tendency. That must be overcome. But it will be more easily overcome if instead of being upset by its presence you detach the inner being from it, rise up above it and view it as a weakness of the lower nature.

*

In a general way the only method of succeeding in having between a man and a woman the free and natural yogic relations that should exist between a sadhak and a sadhika in this Yoga is to be able to meet each other without thinking at all that one is a man and another a woman — both are simply human beings, both sadhaks, both striving to serve the Divine and seeking the Divine alone and none else. Have that fully in yourself and no difficulty is likely to come.

*

All gross animal indulgence of sex desire and impulse would have to be eliminated; it could only continue among those who are not ready for the higher life or not yet ready for a complete spiritual living.

*

It is true that the sex centre and its reactions can be transformed and that an Ananda from above can come down to replace the animal sex reaction. The sex impulse is a degradation of this Ananda.

Speech

Remember the following rules with regard to speech:

(1) Not to allow the impulse of speech to assert itself too much or say anything without reflection, but to speak always with a conscious control and only what is necessary and helpful.

(2) To avoid all debates, dispute or too animated discussion and simply say what has to be said and leave it there. There should also be no insistence that you are right and the others wrong, but what is said should only be thrown in as a contribution to the consideration of the truth of the matter.

(3) To keep the tone of speech and the wording very quiet and calm and uninsistent.

(4) Not to mind at all if others are heated and dispute, but remain quiet and undisturbed and yourself speak only what can help things to be smooth again.

(5) If there is gossip about others and harsh criticism (specially about sadhaks), not to join — for these things are helpful in no way and only lower the consciousness from its higher level.

(6) To avoid all that would hurt or wound others.

*

A gossiping spirit is always an obstacle.

*

Speech is usually the expression of the superficial nature; therefore to throw oneself out too much in such speech wastes the energy and prevents the inward listening which brings the word of true knowledge. "Talk less and gain power" has essentially the same meaning; not only a truer knowledge, but a greater power comes to one in the quietude and silence of the mind.

*

The Mother's warning to you against the undesirability of too much talk, loose chat and gossip, social self-dispersion was entirely meant and stands; when you indulge in these things, you throw yourself out into a very small and ignorant consciousness in which your vital defects get free play and this is likely to bring you out of what you have developed in your inner consciousness.

*

The best way to get mastery over speech and action is to learn to stand back from the outer mind and vital and achieve an inner silence from which one can act on the outer self. If one puts oneself in the true relation with the Mother he will always get help as much as he can receive or use.

*

Dissimulation and falsity of speech is an exceedingly injurious habit of the lower nature. Those who are not straightforward cannot profit by the Mother's help, for they themselves turn it away. Unless they change, they cannot hope for the descent of the Supramental Light and Truth into the lower vital and physical nature; they remain stuck in their own self-created mud and cannot progress.

*

Control of speech is very necessary for the physical change. To minimise speech is sure to be helpful both for right action and for inner sadhana.

*

Speech breaks out as the expression of the vital and its habits, without caring to wait for the control of the mind; the tongue has been spoken of as the unruly member.

*

It is better to be more strict about not talking of others and criticising them with the ordinary mind. It is necessary in order to develop a deeper consciousness and outlook on things that understands in silence the movements of Nature in oneself and others and is not moved or disturbed or superficially interested and drawn into an external movement.

*

The sadhaks of this Ashram are not perfect — they have plenty of weaknesses and wrong movements. It is blindness not to be able to see that; only it should not lead to a criticising or condemnatory attitude towards persons — and it should be regarded as the play of forces which have to be overcome.

*

Yes, excessive hilarity and unnecessary chat do most undoubtedly dissipate the force. A great moderation is necessary in these things.

The Mother:

Be careful always to keep the living Presence and Protection around you when you speak to people, and speak as little as possible.

*

It is the control over oneself that is the first thing needed, and especially the control over one's tongue. If people could learn to keep silent how many troubles would be avoided!

*

It is a much greater and more fruitful austerity to control one's speech than to abolish it altogether. The world is deafened with the noise of his speech and at times you almost seem to miss the harmonious silence of the vegetable kingdom. It is a well-known fact that the less the mental power the greater is the need for speech.

*

If you are not alone and you live with others, cultivate the habit not to throw yourself out constantly into spoken words, you will see little by little that an inner understanding has been established between you and the others; you will then be able to communicate with each other with the minimum speech or no speech at all. This outer silence is very favourable to inner peace and if you have good will and constant aspiration you will be able to create an atmosphere conducive to progress.

You should always control the words you utter and must not

let your tongue be moved by an outburst of anger, violence or temper. It is not merely the quarrel itself which is bad in its results; it is the fact that you lend your tongue for the projection of bad vibrations into the atmosphere, for nothing is more contagious than the vibration of sound. Among the most undesirable kinds of talkativeness should be included all that one says about others. In any case and in a general way, the less one speaks of others, — even if it be in praise of them — the better it is. Already it is so difficult to know exactly what happens in oneself, how to know then with certainty what is happening in others. Refrain then from pronouncing upon any person one of those irrevocable judgments which can only be stupidity, if not malice.

Besides, in the matter of inner life and spiritual effort, the use of speech should be put under a still more stringent rule: nothing should be spoken unless it is absolutely necessary to do so.

VITAL

A weak vital has not the strength to turn spiritually — and being weak, more easily falls under a wrong influence and even when it wants finds it difficult to accept anything beyond its own habitual nature. The strong vital, when the will is there, can do it much more easily.

*

But this must always be remembered that the vital being and the life-force in man are separated from the Divine Light and, so separated, they are an instrument for any power that can take hold of them, illumined or obscure, divine or undivine. It is therefore only when this vital is transformed and made a pure and strong instrument of the Divine Shakti, that there can be a divine life. It must be put in contact with the higher consciousness, it must be surrendered to the true control, it must be placed under the government of the Divine.

*

The vital must not only reject all lower movements, but open and receive the light from above so that it may receive and know the Divine Will and its impulsion — it can then be called enlightened.

The lower vital takes a mean and petty pleasure in picking out the faults of others and thereby one hampers one's own progress and that of the subject of the criticism.

*

But the vital's test is very foolish. If the sadhana goes on whether you see the Mother or not, that would rather show that the psychic connection is permanently there and active always and does not depend on the physical contact. The vital seems to think the sadhana ought to cease if you would not see the Mother but that would only mean that the love and devotion need the stimulus of physical contact. The greatest test of love and devotion is on the contrary when it burns as strongly in long absence as in the presence. If your sadhana went on as well on non-pranam as on Pranam days, it would not prove that love and devotion are not there, but that they are so strong as to be self-existent in all circumstances.

*

There are ranges of consciousness above and below the human range, with which the normal human has no contact and they seem to it unconscious.

*

The vital in its outer form in the ignorance generates the desire-soul which governs most men and which they mistake often for the real soul.

The vital as the desire-soul and desire-nature controls the consciousness to a large extent in most men, because men are governed by desire. It is the mental, vital, physical ego that we take for our being until we get knowledge.

*

Our experience is that too much vital eagerness, too much insistence often blocks the way, it makes a sort of obstructing mass or a whirl of restlessness and disturbance which leaves no quiet space for the Divine to get in. The habit of this vital element starts up and takes hold and interrupts the progress made.

*

When the vital takes the lead, then unrest, despondency, unhappiness can always come, since these things are the very nature of the vital — the vital can never remain constantly in joy and peace, for it needs their opposites in order to have the sense of the drama of life. If the psychic were always there in front, the desert would be no longer a desert and the wilderness would blossom with the rose.

*

There are three obstacles that one has to overcome in the vital and they are very difficult to overcome, lust (sexual desire), wrath and rajasic ego.

*

These vital forces are around everywhere, and if one opens the door to them, they come in wherever you are. One who wants to do sadhana has no business to indulge in such panics; it is a weakness incompatible with the demands of the Yoga and, if one cannot throw it aside, it is safer not to try the Yoga. Each victory gained over oneself means new strength to gain more victories.

When some weakness comes up you should take it as an opportunity to know what is still to be done and call down the strength into that part.

*

One cannot take advantage of any help given him because his vital nature cherishes its weakness and is always indulging and rhetorically expressing it instead of throwing it away with contempt as a thing unworthy of manhood and unfit for a sadhak. It is only if he so rejects it that he can receive strength and stand in life or progress in the sadhana. This is a temperament which the gods will not help because they know that help is useless, for it will either not be received or will be spilled and wasted.

*

It is this idea that you are helpless because the vital consents to the wrong movement that comes in the way. You have to put your inner will and the Mother's light on the vital so that it shall change, not leave it to do what it likes. The Mother's force can act, but on condition that the assent of the being is there.

*

The human vital is almost always of that nature; it is by the use of the mental will that they discipline it, compelling it to do not what it wants but what the reason or the will sees to be right or desirable. In Yoga one uses the inner will and compels the vital to submit itself to tapasya so that it may become calm, strong, obedient. The vital is a good instrument but a bad master. If you allow it to follow its likes and dislikes, its fancies, its desires, its bad habits, it becomes your master and peace and happiness are no longer possible.

*

Put the Mother's notice henceforth at the door of your vital being, "No falsehood hereafter shall ever enter here," and station a sentry there to see that it is put into execution.

*

The lower vital has its place, it is not to be crushed or killed, but it has to be changed, "caught hold of by both ends", at the upper end a master and control, at the lower end a right use. The main thing is to get rid of attachment and desire; it is then that an entirely right use becomes possible.

*

It is better to be a stone on the road to the Divine than soft and weak clay in the muddy paths of the ordinary vital human nature.

*

The vital is too selfish to have any gratitude. The more it gets the more it demands and it takes everything as its right and every denial of what it wants as an injustice and an offence.

The unregenerate vital in the average human nature is not grateful for a benefit, it resents being under an obligation. So long as the benefit continues, it is effusive and says sweet things, as soon as it expects nothing more it turns round and bites the hands that fed it. Sometimes it does that even before, when it thinks it can do it without the benefactor knowing the origin of the slander, fault-finding or abuse. In all these dealings, of course, people with a developed psychic element are by nature grateful and do not behave in this way.

SECTION TWO

ART

If Art's service is but to imitate Nature, then burn all the picture galleries and let us have instead photographic studios. It is because Art reveals what Nature hides that a small picture is worth more than all the jewels of the millionaires and the treasures of the princes.

If you only imitate visible Nature, you will perpetrate either a corpse, a dead sketch or a monstrosity; Truth lives in that which goes behind and beyond the visible and sensible.

*

It is wrong to measure the greatness of any art like that. Each of the great arts has its own appeal and its own way of appeal and each in its own way is supreme above all others.

*

But great art is not satisfied with representing the intellectual truth of things, which is always their superficial or exterior truth; it seeks for a deeper and original truth which escapes the eye of the mere sense or the mere reason, the soul in them, the unseen reality which is not that of their form and process but of their spirit.... Always the truth it seeks is first and foremost the truth of beauty, — not, again, the formal beauty alone or the beauty of proportion and right process which is what the sense and the reason seek, but the soul of beauty which is hidden from the ordinary eye and the ordinary mind and revealed in its fullness only to the unsealed vision of the poet and artist in man who can seize the secret significances of the universal poet and artist, the divine creator who dwells as their soul and spirit in the forms he has created.

The Mother:

Art is a means, not an end; it is a means of expression. The personality of an artist counts no longer; he is an agent, a channel, his art a means of expressing his relations with the Divine. If you consider it in this light, art is not very different from Yoga.

In India all her architecture, her sculpture, her painting have proceeded from this source and were inspired by this ideal. If they are true artists and try to see beyond and use their art for the expression of the inner world, they grow in consciousness by their concentration on the subject. But most of those who call themselves artists draw their inspiration from the vital world only; and it carries in it no high or great significance.

ASHRAM LIFE

This Ashram has been created with another object than that ordinarily common to such institutions, not for the renunciation of the world but as a centre and a field of practice for the evolution of another kind and form of life which would in the final end be moved by a higher spiritual consciousness and embody a greater life of the spirit.

This is not an Ashram like others — the members are not Sanyasis; it is not Moksha that is the sole aim of the Yoga here. What is being done here is a preparation for a work — a work which will be founded on Yogic consciousness and Yoga-Shakti, and can have no other foundation.

*

A sadhaka in the Ashram is expected to observe the following conditions:

All physical sexual relation or connection between a sadhak and sadhika are absolutely forbidden and inadmissible in the Ashram.

All vital relations of a sexual character are contrary to the sadhana and must also be given up by those who wish to stay in the Ashram and progress in the Yoga.

Even a husband and wife must stop all conjugal relations and regard each other as fellow-sadhaks only and not as husband and wife. It is not as man and woman that the sadhaks are here; they have not come here to continue or to form vital or physical sexual relations between themselves under any pretext but to practise Yoga.

Any sadhak forming vital relations with others under the pretext of a psychic or spiritual relation is deceiving himself and violating the Truth and breaking the rule of the Yoga.

No sadhak should worship another sadhak or look on him as the embodied Divine; such movements are contrary to the sadhana and to the discipline of the Ashram and create false movements in the atmosphere.

*

You are not yet ready or fit as yet for life in the Ashram. There are certain weaknesses of the adhara (especially of the vital nature and the physical mind) which must be got rid of before you should think of joining the Ashram. To practise Yoga, as a member of the Ashram is to push yourself into the centre of a pressure for transformation of the whole being and, especially just now, of the physical mind and the lower vital nature, which that mind in you and your nervous parts in their present impurity and weakness might not be able to bear. It is our repeated experience that those who have this weakness are better outside the Ashram where they can slowly prepare and purify themselves without any premature pressure.

*

The Mother and I are equal. Also she is supreme here and has the right to arrange the work as she thinks best for the work, no one has any right or claim or proprietorship over any work that may be given to him. The Ashram is the Mother's creation and would not have existed but for her, the work she does is her creation and has not been given to her and cannot be taken from her. Try to understand this elementary truth, if you want to have any right relation or attitude towards the Mother.

*

There are only two possible foundations for the material life here. One is that one is a member of an Ashram founded on the principle of self-giving and surrender. One belongs to the Divine and all one has belongs to the Divine; in giving one gives not what is one's own but what already belongs to the Divine. There is no question of payment or return, no bargain, no room for demand and desire. The Mother is in sole charge and arranges things as best they can be arranged within the means at her disposal and the capacities of her instruments. She is under no obligation to act according to the mental standards or vital desires and claims of the sadhaks; she is not obliged to use a democratic equality in her dealings with them.

The Mother:

The usual Sadhanas have for their aim union with the Supreme Consciousness (Sat-chit-ananda). And they who reach there, are satisfied with their own liberation and leave the world to its unhappy plight. On the contrary, Sri Aurobindo's Sadhana starts where the others end. Once the union with the Supreme is realised, one must bring down that realisation to the external world and change the conditions of life upon the earth until a total transformation is accomplished. In accordance with this aim, the Sadhaks of the integral Yoga do not retire from the world to lead a life of contemplation and meditation.

*

Don't judge on appearances and do not listen to what people say, because these two things are misleading.

There is in the Ashram no exterior discipline and no visible test. But the inner test is severe and constant, one must be very sincere in the aspiration to surmount all egoism and to conquer all vanity in order to be able to stay here. A complete surrender is not outwardly exacted but it is indispensable for those who wish to stick on, and many things come to test the sincerity of this surrender. However, the Grace and the help are always there for those who aspire for them and their power is limitless when received with faith and confidence.

BEAUTY

Beauty is as much an expression of the Divine as Knowledge, Power or Ananda. Does any one ask why does the Mother want to manifest the divine consciousness by knowledge or by power and not by ignorance and weakness? It would not be a more absurd or meaningless question than the one put by the vital against her wearing artistic and beautiful dress. Is it your notion that the Divine should be represented on earth by poverty and ugliness?

Outer things are the expression of something in the inner reality. A fine sari or a palace are expressions of the principle of beauty in things and that is their main value. The Divine Consciousness is not bound by these things and has no attachment, but it is also not bound to abstain from them if beauty in things is part of its intended action. The Mother, when the Ashram was still unformed, was wearing patched cotton saris. When she took up the work, it was necessary to change her habits, so she did so.

*

To find highest beauty is to find God; to reveal, to embody, to create as we say, highest beauty is to bring out of our souls the living image and power of God.

The Mother:

It is one of the greatest weapons of the Asura at work when you are taught to shun beauty. It has been the ruin of India. The Divine manifests in the psychic as love, in the mind as knowledge, in the vital as power and in the physical as beauty. If you discard beauty it means that you are depriving the Divine of his manifestation in the material and you hand over that part to the Asura.

*

In the physical world, of all things it is beauty that expresses best the Divine. The physical world is the world of forms and the perfection of forms is beauty. Beauty interprets, expresses, manifests the Eternal. Its role is to put all manifested nature in contact with the Eternal through the perfection of form, through harmony and a sense of the ideal which uplifts and leads towards something higher.

CONSCIOUSNESS

The higher consciousness is a concentrated consciousness, concentrated in the Divine Unity and in the working out of the Divine Will, not dispersed and rushing about after this or that mental idea or vital desire or physical need as in the ordinary human consciousness — also not invaded by a hundred haphazard thoughts, feelings and impulses, but master of itself, centred and harmonious.

In the externalised consciousness obscurity and suffering can always be there; the more the internalised consciousness reigns, the more these things are pushed back and out, and with the full internalised consciousness they cannot remain.

*

There are always two different consciousnesses in the human being, one outward in which he ordinarily lives, the other inward and concealed of which he knows nothing. When one does sadhana, the inner consciousness begins to open and one is able to go inside and have all kinds of experiences there. As the sadhana progresses, one begins to live more and more in this inner being and the outer becomes more and more superficial. At first the inner consciousness seems to be the dream and the outer the waking reality. Afterwards the inner consciousness becomes the reality and the outer is felt by many as a dream or delusion, or else something superficial and external. The inner consciousness begins to be a place of deep peace, light, happiness, love, closeness to the Divine or the presence of the Divine, the Mother. One is then aware of two consciousnesses, the inner one and the outer which has to be changed into its counterpart and instrument — that also must become full of peace, light, union with the Divine.

*

To be too much occupied in mind with the outer difficulties keeps the consciousness externalised. Living inwardly you will find the Mother close to you and realise her will and her action.

*

All that exists or can exist in this or any other universe can be rendered into terms of consciousness; there is nothing that cannot be known. This knowing need not be always a mental knowledge. For the greater part of existence is either above or below mind, and mind can know only indirectly what is above or what is below it. But the one true and complete way of knowing is by direct knowledge.

The Unmanifested Supreme is beyond all definition and description by mind or speech; no definition the mind can make, affirmative or negative, which can be at all expressive of it or adequate.

DARSHANS, BLESSINGS

There is the utility of the physical approach to the Mother — the approach of the embodied mind and vital to her embodied Power. In her universal action the Mother acts according to the law of things — in her embodied physical action is the opportunity of a constant Grace — it is for that the embodiment takes place.

The Divine Mother is the Consciousness and Force of the Divine — which is the Mother of all things.

It is certainly quite true that the psychic contact can exist at a distance and that the Divine is not limited by place, but is everywhere. It is not necessary for everybody to be in the Ashram or physically near the Mother in order to lead the spiritual life or to practise the Yoga, especially in its early stages. But it is only one side of the truth; there is another, otherwise the logical conclusion might be that there was no necessity for the Mother to be here at all, or for the existence of the Ashram, or for anyone to come here.

The psychic being is there in all, but in very few it is well developed, well built up in the consciousness or prominent in the front; in most it is veiled, often ineffective or only an influence, not conscious enough or strong enough to support the spiritual life. It is for this reason that it is necessary for those drawn towards this Truth to come here in order that they may receive the touch which will bring about or prepare the awakening of the psychic being — that is for them the beginning of the effective psychic contact.

When the touch has been given or the development effected, so far as the sadhak is at the moment capable of it, he returns to the outside world and under the protection and guidance even at a distance is able to keep the contact and go on with his spiritual life. But the influences of the outside world are not favourable to the psychic contact and the psychic development and, if the sadhak is not sufficiently careful or concentrated, the psychic contact may easily be lost after a time or get covered over and the development may become retarded, stationary or even diminished by adverse movements or influences. It is for that the necessity exists and is often felt of a return to the place of the central influence in order to fortify or recover the contact or to restore or give a fresh forward impulse to the development.

The physical nearness to the Mother is indispensable for the fullness of the sadhana on the physical plane. Transformation of the physical and external being is not possible otherwise.

*

The right attitude to approach the Mother when she sees one is to keep the being perfectly quiet and open to receive, without any activity of the mind or desire in the vital, with only the surrender and the psychic readiness to accept whatever is given.

The physical contact of the Mother means for her an interchange, a pouring out of her forces and a receiving of things good, bad and mixed from them which often involves a great labour of adjustment and elimination, and in many cases, a severe strain on the body.

The best way for Darshan is to keep oneself very collected and quiet and open to receive whatever the Mother gives.

*

During Darshan and Blessings, the time has nothing to do with it. One hour's touch or a moment's touch — as much can be given by the one as by the other. The Mother gives in both ways. Through the eyes it is to the psychic, through the hand to the material.

It is when the Mother puts her force into the flower that it becomes more than a symbol. It then can become very effective if there is receptivity in the one who receives.

DEATH AND REBIRTH

The soul takes birth each time, and each time a mind, life and body are formed out of the materials of universal Nature, according to the soul's past evolution and its need for the future. When the body is dissolved after death, the vital goes into the vital plane and remains there for a time, but after a time the vital sheath disappears. The last to dissolve is the mental sheath. Finally the soul or psychic being retires into the psychic world to rest there till a new birth is close.

The soul gathers the essential elements of its experiences in life and makes that its basis of growth in the evolution; when it returns to birth it takes up with its mental, vital, physical sheaths so much of its Karma as is useful to it in the new life for farther experience.

It is really for the vital part of the being that Sraddha and rites are done — to help the being to get rid of the vital vibrations which still attach it to the earth or to the vital worlds, so that it may pass quickly to its rest in the psychic peace.

*

The soul comes into birth for experience, for growth, for evolution till it can bring the Divine into matter. It is the central being that incarnates, not the outer personality — the personality is simply a mould that it creates for its figures of experience in that one life. In another birth it will create for itself a different personality, different capacities, a different life and career.

It is not the personality, the character that is of the first importance in rebirth — it is the psychic being who stands behind the evolution of the nature and evolves with it. The psychic when it departs from the body, shedding even the mental and vital on its way to its resting place, carries with it the heart of its experiences. That is the permanent addition, it is that that helps in the growth towards the Divine.

*

Death is there because the being in the body is not yet developed enough to go on growing in the same body without the need of change and the body itself is not sufficiently conscious. If the mind and vital and the body itself were more conscious and plastic, death would not be necessary.

*

At the time of death the being goes out of the body through the head; it goes out in the subtle body and goes to different planes of existence for a short time until it has gone through certain experiences which are the result of its earthly existence. Afterwards it reaches the psychic world where it rests in a kind of sleep, until it is time for it to start a new life on earth. That is what happens usually — but there are some beings who are more developed and do not follow this course.

*

The soul does not go back to animal condition; but a part of the vital personality may disjoin itself and join an animal birth to work out its animal propensities there.

There is after death a period in which one passes through the vital world and lives there for a time. It is only the first part of this transit that can be dangerous or painful. One can help departed souls by one's good will or by occult means, if one has the knowledge. The one thing that one should not do is to hold them back by sorrow for them or longing or by anything else that would pull them nearer to earth or delay their journey to their place of rest.

*

Usually, a soul follows continuously the same line of sex. If there are shiftings of sex, it is, as a rule, a matter of parts of the personality which are not central.

*

No rule can be laid with regard to what time the psychic being joins the new body, for these circumstances vary with the individual. Some psychic beings get into relation with the birth-environment and the parents from the time of inception and determine the preparation of the personality and future in the embryo, others join only at the time of delivery, others even later on in the life and in these cases it is some emanation of the psychic being which upholds the life. It should be noted that the conditions of the future birth are determined fundamentally not during the stay in the psychic world but at the time of death — the psychic being then chooses what it should work out in the next terrestrial appearance and the conditions arrange themselves accordingly.

*

Note that the idea of rebirth and the circumstances of the new life as a reward or punishment for punya or papa is a crude human idea of "justice" which is quite unphilosophical and unspiritual and distorts the true intention of life. Life here is an evolution and the soul grows by experience, working out by it this or that in the nature, and if there is suffering, it is for the purpose of that working out, not as a judgment inflicted by God or Cosmic Law on the errors or stumblings which are inevitable in the Ignorance.

*

But the soul, the psychic being, once having reached the human consciousness cannot go back to the inferior animal consciousness any more than it can go back into a tree or an ephemeral insect. What is true is that some part of the vital energy or the formed instrumental consciousness or nature can and very frequently does so, if it is strongly attached to anything in the earth life. This may account for some cases of immediate rebirth with full memory in human forms also. Ordinarily, it is only by Yogic development or by clairvoyance that the exact memory of past lives can be brought back.

The psychic does not give up the mental and other sheaths immediately at death. It is said that it takes three years on the whole to get clear away from the zone of communicability with the earth — though there may be cases of slower or quicker passage.

*

All kinds of work are equal before the Divine and all men have the same Brahman within them is one truth, but that development is not equal in all is another. The idea that it needs a special punya to be born as a Bhangi is, of course, one of these forceful exaggerations of an idea which are common with the Mahatma and impress greatly the mind of his hearers. But obviously the cultural development is more valuable than the service of the physical needs for the progress of humanity as opposed to its first static condition, and that development can even lead to the minimising and perhaps the entire disappearance by scientific inventions of the need of the functions of the scavenger. In any case, it is not true that the Bhangi life is superior to the Brahmin life and the reward of a special righteousness. On the other hand, the traditional conception that a man is superior to others because he is born a Brahmin is not rational or justifiable.

The Mother:

In rebirth it is only the psychic being that passes from body to body. Logically, then neither the mental nor the vital being can remember past lives or recognise itself in the character of mode of life of this or that person. The psychic being alone can remember; and it is by becoming conscious of our psychic being that we can have at the same time exact impressions about our past lives.

DISCIPLINE

This constant disobedience and indiscipline is a radical obstacle to the sadhana and the worst possible example to others.

*

It is a deficiency of psychic perception and spiritual discrimination that makes people to ignore the importance of obedience. It is the mind wanting to follow its own way of thinking and the vital seeking freedom for its desires. The obedience is necessary so as to get away from one's own mind and vital and learn to follow the Truth.

*

The discipline has been laid down (in the Ashram) by the Mother — to break it is disobedience to the Divine.

*

It is when you are free from the lower Nature that Mother's will is the Law. When subject to the lower Nature, the lower Nature is constantly disobeying the Divine Will.

DOCTORS AND DISEASES

The Mother and I have no preference for allopathy. The Mother thinks doctors very usually make things worse instead of better by spoiling Nature's resistance to illness by excessive and ill-directed use of their medicines.

Medical Science has been more a curse to mankind than a blessing. It has weakened the natural health of man and multiplied individual diseases; it has implanted fear and dependence in the mind and body; it has taught our health to repose not on natural soundness but a rickety and distasteful witch compact from the mineral and vegetable kingdom.

It is not the medicine that cures so much as the patient's faith in the doctor and the medicine. Both are a clumsy substitute for the natural faith in one's own self-power which they have themselves destroyed.

The healthiest ages of mankind were those in which there were the fewest material remedies. We ought to use the divine health in us to cure and prevent diseases.

Health protected by twenty-thousand precautions is the gospel of the doctors; but it is not God's evangel for the body, nor Nature's.

Man was once naturally healthy and could revert to that primal condition if he were suffered; but Medical Science pursues our body with an innumerable pack of drugs and assails the imagination with ravening hordes of microbes.

It should take long for self-cure to replace medicine; because of the fear, self-distrust and unnatural physical reliance on drugs which Medical Science has taught to our minds and bodies and made our second nature.

Distrust of the curative power within us was our physical fall from Paradise. Medical Science and a bad heredity are the two angels of God who stand at the gates to forbid our return and re-entry.

EDUCATION

It is true of every soul on earth that it is a portion of the Divine Mother passing through the experiences of the Ignorance in order to arrive at the truth of its being and be the instrument of a Divine Manifestation and work here. The body is meant for keeping the Divine consciousness linked to the physical world.

*

I think I made it clear ... that sport was not sadhana, that it belonged to what I called the lower end of things, but that it might be used not merely for amusement or recreation or the maintenance of health, but for a greater efficiency of the body and for the development of certain qualities and capacities, not of the body only but of morale and discipline and the stimulation of mental energies: but I pointed out also that these could be and were developed by other means and that there were limitations to this utility. In fact, it is only by sadhana that one could go beyond the limits natural to the lower end means....

For the immediate object of my endeavours is to establish spiritual life on earth and for that the first necessity must always be to realise the Divine; only then can life be spiritualised or what I have called the Life Divine be made possible; the creation of something that could be called a divine body could be only an ulterior aim undertaken as part of this transformation.

We do not want only sportsmen in the Ashram: that would make it not an Ashram but a playground. The sports and physical exercises are primarily for the children of the school. The younger sadhaks are allowed, not enjoined or even recommended, to join in these sports, but certainly they are not supposed to be sportsmen only: they have other and more important things to do.... In the old Ashrams the boys and young men who were brought up in them were trained in many things belonging to life. ... To concentrate most on one's own spiritual growth and experience is the first necessity of the sadhak.

*

The first principle of true teaching is that nothing can be taught.

The teacher is not an instructor or task-master, he is a helper and a guide. His business is to suggest and not to impose. He does not actually train the pupil's mind, he only shows him how to perfect his instruments of knowledge and helps and encourages him in the process. He does not impart knowledge to him, he shows him how to acquire knowledge for himself. The idea of hammering the child into the shape desired by the parent or teacher is a barbarous and ignorant superstition. It is a selfish tyranny over a human soul and a wound to a nation, which loses the benefit of the best that a man could have given it. The chief aim of education should be to help the growing soul to draw out that in itself which is best and make it perfect for a noble use. A free and natural growth is the condition of genuine development.

*

The only way for him to train himself morally is to habituate himself to the right emotions, the noblest associations, the best mental, emotional and physical habits and the following out in right action of the fundamental impulses of his essential nature. You can impose a certain discipline on children, dress them into a certain mould, lash them into a desired path, but unless you can get their hearts and natures on your side, the conformity to this imposed rule becomes a hypocritical and heartless, a conventional, often a cowardly compliance.

The first rule of moral training is to suggest and invite, not command or impose.

The thirst of knowledge, the self-devotion, the purity, the renunciation of the Brahmin, — the courage, the ardour, honour, nobility, chivalry, patriotism of the Kshatriya, — the beneficence, skill, industry, generous enterprise and large open-handedness of the Vaishya, — the self-effacement and loving service of the Sudra, — these are the qualities of the Aryan. They constitute the moral temper we desire in our young men in the whole nation. But how can we get them if we do not give opportunities to the young to train themselves in the Aryan tradition?

*

Wildness and recklessness of many young natures are only the overflowings of an excessive strength, greatness and nobility. They should be purified, not discouraged.

*

Religion has to be lived, not learned as a creed. No religious teaching is of any value unless it is lived, and the use of various kinds of Sadhana, spiritual self-training and exercise is the only effective preparation for religious living.

*

Every child is an inquirer, an investigator, an analyser, a merciless anatomist. Appeal to those qualities in him and let him acquire without knowing it the right temper and the necessary fundamental knowledge of the scientist. Every child has an insatiable intellectual curiosity and turn for metaphysical enquiry. Use it to draw him on slowly to an understanding of the world and himself.

*

It is by allowing Nature to work that we get the benefit of the gifts she has bestowed on us. Humanity in its education of children has chosen to thwart and hamper her processes and, by so doing, has done much to thwart and hamper the rapidity of its onward march.

The Mother:

An aimless life is always a miserable life. Everyone should have an aim. But do not forget that on the quality of your aim will depend the quality of your life. Your aim should be high and wide, generous and disinterested; this will make your life precious to yourself and to all.

But whatever your ideal, it cannot be perfectly realised unless you have realised perfection in yourself; and to work for your perfection the first step is to become conscious of yourself, of the different parts of your being and their respective activities.

In its natural state the human mind is always limited in its vision, narrow in its understanding, rigid in its conceptions, and a certain effort is needed to enlarge it.

Knowledge belongs to a region much higher than that of the human mind. The mind has to be made silent and attentive in order to receive knowledge from above and manifest it.

The education of a human being should begin at his very birth and continue throughout the whole length of his life; and the education to be complete must have five principal aspects: the physical, the vital, the mental, the psychic and the spiritual.

*

The first thing to do in order to be able to educate the child, is to educate oneself, to become conscious and master of oneself so that one does not set a bad example to one's child. For it is through example that education becomes effective. To say good words, give wise advice to a child has very little effect, if one does not show by one's living example the truth of what one teaches.

*

If you wish to be respected by your child, have respect for yourself and be at every moment worthy of respect. Never be arbitrary, despotic, impatient, ill-tempered. When your child asks you a question, do not answer him by a stupidity or a foolishness, under the pretext that he cannot understand you.

*

Do not scold your child except with a definite purpose and only when quite indispensable. A child too often scolded gets hardened to rebuke and comes to attach little importance to words or severity of tone. Particularly, take care not to rebuke him for a fault which you yourself commit.

... When a child has made a mistake, see that he confesses it to you spontaneously and frankly; and when he has confessed, make him understand with kindness and affection what was wrong in his movement and that he should not repeat it. In any case, never scold him; a fault confessed must be forgiven. You should not allow any fear to slip in between you and your child; fear is a disastrous way to education.

... If the child, from the very beginning of his existence, takes to good habits, that will save him a good deal of trouble and inconvenience during the whole of his life. Bad habits are formed too early and too quickly that may have disastrous consequences for the whole life.

... He must avoid, in his daily food, all that merely stuffs and causes heaviness; particularly, he must be taught to eat according to his hunger, neither more or less, and not to make food an occasion to satisfy his greed and gluttony. From one's very childhood, one should know that one eats in order to give to the body strength and health, and not to enjoy the pleasures of the palate.

... It is not fair to demand services from a child, as if it is his duty to serve his parents. The contrary would be more true: certainly it is natural that parents should serve their children, at least take great care of them. It is only if the child chooses freely to work for the family and does the work as a play that the thing is admissible.

... The child must be shown, made to appreciate, taught to love beautiful, lofty, healthy and noble things, whether in nature or in human creation. The sovereign means is to rouse in the child interest in the thing that one wishes to teach, the taste for work, the will to progress. To love to learn is the most precious gift that one can make to a child; to love to learn always and everywhere.

... Studies strengthen the mind and turn the attention from concentrating on the impulses and desires of the vital. Concentrating on studies is one of the most powerful means of controlling the mind and the vital; that is why it is so important to study.

... If the power of concentration and attention is continuously cultivated, the active external consciousness will allow only those thoughts that are needed and then they become all the more dynamic and effective. And if, in the intensity of concentration, it is necessary not to think at all, all mental vibration can be stopped and an almost total silence secured. In this silence one can open gradually to the higher mental regions and learn to record the inspirations that come from there.

The art of giving rest to one's mind is a thing to be acquired. Changing mental activity is a way of rest; but the greatest possible rest lies in silence.

*

Every human being carries hidden within him the possibility of a greater consciousness beyond the frame of his normal life through which he can participate in a higher and vaster life. What the human mind does not know and cannot do, this consciousness knows and does.

*

The first and most important point which must never be forgotten is that with the mind it is impossible to judge of spiritual things. All who have written on yogic discipline have said so, but very few are those who put it into practice and yet, in order to proceed on the path, it is absolutely indispensable to abstain from all mental judgment, mental opinion and reaction.

*

Give up all personal seeking for comfort, satisfaction, enjoyment or happiness. Be only a burning fire for progress, take whatever comes to you as a help for progress and make at once the progress required.

Try to take pleasure in all you do, but never do anything for the sake of pleasure. Never get excited, nervous or agitated. Remain perfectly quiet in the face of anything and everything. And yet be always awake to find out the progress you have still to make and lose no time in making it.

*

The Vital in man's nature, is a despotic and exacting tyrant. It is a master that is satisfied by nothing and its demands have no limit. The conviction that makes one believe that one has the right to be happy leads, as a matter of course, towards the will to live one's life at any cost. This attitude in its obscure and aggressive egoism brings about every conflict and misery, deception and discouragement, ending often in a catastrophe.

In the world, as it actually is, the goal of life is not to secure personal happiness, but to awaken the individual progressively towards the truth-consciousness.

*

The spiritual consciousness means to live the infinite and eternal, to throw oneself outside all creation, beyond time and space. To become fully aware of your psychic being and to live a psychic life you must abolish in you all selfishness; but to live a spiritual life you must be selfless.

EVOLUTION

A progressive evolution of the visible and invisible instruments of the Spirit is the whole law of the earth nature. Spirit has concealed itself in inconscient matter. It evolves into forms of matter by the working of matter forces. It is only when this has been sufficiently done, that it thinks of life. A subconscient life and its imprisoned forces were there all the time in matter and its forces. Afterwards came an evolution of mind in many forms by the working of liberated mind-forces. In those life-forces in matter and even in the very substance of matter mind was latent. An evolution of mind in the living form by a working of liberated mind-force was the third chapter of the story. The third chapter is not completed, neither will it be the end of the narrative.

The evolution of the earth-nature is not finished because it has manifested only three powers out of the seven-fold scale of consciousness that is involved in manifested Nature. It has brought out from its apparent inconscience only the three powers of Mind and Life and Matter.

*

The supramental change is a thing decreed and inevitable in the evolution of the earth-consciousness; for its upward ascent is not ended and mind is not its last summit.

*

The earth is a material field of evolution. Mind and Life, Supermind, Sachchidananda are in principle involved there in the earth-consciousness; but only matter is at first organised; then life descends from the life plane and gives shape and organisation and activity to the life principle in matter, creates the plant and animal; then mind descends from the mind plane, creating man. Now Supermind is to descend so as to create a supramental race.

*

The Prakriti itself is divided into lower and higher, — the lower is the Prakriti of the Ignorance, the Prakriti of mind, life and matter separated in consciousness from the Divine; the higher is the Divine Prakriti of Sachchidananda with its manifesting power of Supermind, always aware of the Divine and free from Ignorance and its consequences. Man so long as he is in the ignorance is subject to the lower Prakriti, but by spiritual evolution he becomes aware of the higher Nature and seeks to come into contact with it.

*

The material world has evolved life in obedience to a pressure from the vital plane, mind in obedience to a pressure from the mental plane. It is now trying to evolve supermind in obedience to a pressure from the supramental plane.

*

It is something new that has manifested here and it is that that makes the creation worth while. What for instance would be the utility of a supramental creation on earth if it were just the same thing as a supramental creation on the supramental plane? It is that, in principle, but yet something else, a triumphant new self-discovery of the Divine in conditions that are not elsewhere.

*

Out of this apparent Inconscience each potentiality is revealed in its turn, first organised Matter concealing the indwelling Spirit, the Life emerging in the plant and associated in the animal with a growing Mind, the Mind itself evolved and organised in Man. This evolution, this spiritual progression — does it stop short here in the imperfect mental being called Man? In this vision each stage of evolution appears as due to the descent of a higher and higher Power of consciousness, raising the terrestrial level, creating a new stratum, but the highest yet remain to descend and it is by their descent that the riddle of terrestrial existence will receive its solution and not only the soul but Nature herself find her deliverance....

Division, ego, the imperfect consciousness and groping and struggle of a separate self-affirmation are the efficient causes of the suffering and ignorance of this world. Once consciousnesses separated from the one consciousness, they fell inevitably into Ignorance and the last result of Ignorance was Inconscience; from a dark immense Inconscient this material world arises and out of it a soul that by evolution is struggling into consciousness, attracted towards the hidden Light, ascending but still blindly towards the lost Divinity from which it came....

It is by entering into that greater consciousness alone that one can grasp the inevitability of its self-creation and its purpose. To rise to that height of liberation is the true way out and the only means of the indubitable knowledge....

But that liberation and transcendence need not necessarily impose a disappearance, a sheer dissolving cut from the manifestation; it can prepare a liberation into action of the highest Knowledge and an intensity of Power that can transform the world and fulfil the evolutionary urge. It is an ascent from which there is no longer a fall but a winged or self-sustained descent of light, force and Ananda....

As long as the outward personality we call ourselves is centred in the lower powers of consciousness, the riddle of its own existence, its purpose, its necessity is to it an insoluble enigma....

It is only by rising towards a higher consciousness beyond the line and therefore superconscient now to him that he can emerge from his inability and his ignorance. His full liberation and enlightenment will come when he crosses the line into the light of a new super-conscient existence....

But this crossing of the line if turned not only to an ascending but to a descending purpose would mean the transformation of the line from what it now is, a lid, a barrier, into a passage for the higher powers of consciousness of the Being now above it. It would mean a new creation on earth, a bringing in of the ultimate powers which would reverse the conditions here in as much as that would produce a creation raised into the full flood of spiritual and supramental light in place of one emerging into a half-light of mind out of a darkness of material inconscience....

*

If the redemption of the soul from the physical vesture be the object, then there is no need of supramentalisation. Spiritual Mukti and Nirvana are sufficient. If the object is to rise to supraphysical planes, then also there is no need of supramentalisation. One can enter into some heaven above by devotion to the Lord of that heaven. But that is no progression. The other worlds are typal worlds, each fixed in its own kind and type and law. Evolution takes place on the earth and therefore the earth is the proper field for progression. The beings of the other worlds do not progress from one world to another. They remain fixed to their own type.

*

In a general way, a life is only one brief episode in a long history of spiritual evolution in which the soul follows the curve of the line set for the earth, passing through many lives to complete it. It is an evolution out of material inconscience to consciousness and towards the Divine Consciousness, from ignorance to Divine Knowledge, from darkness through half-light to Light, from death to Immortality, from suffering to the Divine Bliss. Suffering is due first to the Ignorance, secondly to the separation of the individual consciousness from the Divine Consciousness and Being, a separation created by the Ignorance — when that ceases, when one lives in the Divine and no more in one's separated smaller self, then only suffering can altogether cease.

*

With regards Supramental, what is more likely to happen is that the principle will be established in the evolution by the descent just as the mental principle was established by the appearance of thinking Mind and Man in earthly life. There will be a race of supramental beings on the earth just as now there is a race of mental beings. Man himself will find a greater possibility of rising to the planes intermediary between his mind and Supermind and making their powers effective in his life, which will mean a great change in humanity on earth.

*

One should not attach too much importance to the life of the body. The body is only an incident in the progress of the soul. Evolution of the soul is the objective of Karmic existence. When one has realised the soul, knowledge and enlightenment come and all the problems are solved. But before that, one should try to get peace, calm and light.

*

The human being on earth is God playing at humanity in a world of matter under the conditions of a hampered density with the ulterior intention of imposing law of spirit on matter and nature of deity upon human nature. Evolution is nothing but the progressive unfolding of Spirit out of the density of material consciousness and the gradual self-revelation of God out of this apparent animal being. Yoga is the application, for this process of divine self-revelation.

The Mother:

As Nature has already created upon earth a mental being, even so, there is now a concentrated activity to bring forth in this mentality a supramental consciousness and individuality. We have here the peerless privilege of being at the very centre of the radiating light, at the source of the force of transformation.

*

Sri Aurobindo incarnated in a human body the supramental consciousness and has not only revealed to us the nature of the path to follow and the method of following it so as to arrive at the goal, but has also by his own personal realisation given us the example; he has provided us, so to say, the proof that the thing can be done and the time is now to do it.

EXPERIENCES — VISIONS

The more intense the experiences that come, the higher the forces that descend, the greater become the possibilities of deviation and error. For the very intensity and the very height of the force excites and aggrandises the movements of the lower nature and raises up in it all opposing elements in their full force, but often in the disguise of truth, wearing a mask of plausible justification. There is needed a great patience, calm, sobriety, balance, an impersonal detachment and sincerity free from all taint of ego or personal human desire. There must be no attachment to any idea of one's own, to any experience, to any kind of imagination, mental building or vital demand; the light of discrimination must always play to detect those things, however fair or plausible they may seem. Otherwise, the Truth will have no chance of establishing itself in its purity in the nature.

*

It would be a great mistake to interfere with the images rising in you. It does not matter whether they are mental or psychic. One must have experience not only of the true psychic, but of the inner mental, inner vital and subtle physical worlds or planes of consciousness. The occurrences of the images is a sign that these are opening and to inhibit them would mean to inhibit the expansion of consciousness and experience without which this Yoga cannot be done.

*

Inner vision is vivid like actual sight, always precise and contains a truth in it. The inner vision can see objects, but it can see instead the vibration of the forces which act through the object. The mental visions are meant to bring in the mind the influence of the things they represent. The cosmic vision is the seeing of the universal movements — it has nothing to do with the psychic necessarily.

*

The human mind's activities come very much in the way of receiving the higher knowledge. During the experience the mind should be quiet. After the experience is over it can be active. If it is active while it is there, the experience may stop altogether. The attempt of the mind and vital to seize on the experience is always one of the chief obstacles.

*

One of the first needs in our Yoga is a discrimination and a psychic tact distinguishing the false from the true, putting each thing in its place and giving it its true value or absence of value, not carried away by the excitement of the mind or the vital being.

*

It is not usually good to tell the experiences to others. It weakens the experience and tends to bring down the consciousness.

*

Telling of one's own experiences to others is very much discouraged by most Yogis — they say it is harmful to the sadhana. I have certainly seen and heard of any number of instances in which people were having a flow of experiences and, when they told, the flow was lost. I suppose however it ceases to apply after one has reached a certain long-established stability in the experience, that is to say when the experience amounts to a definite and permanent realisation, something finally and irrevocably added to the consciousness.

*

The consciousness from which these experiences come is always there pressing to bring them in. The reason why they don't come in freely or stay is the activity of the mind and vital always rushing about thinking this, wanting that, trying to perform mountaineering feats on all the hillocks of the lower nature instead of nourishing a strong and simple aspiration and opening to the higher consciousness that it may come in and do its own work.

*

Experiences come first in this isolated way, afterwards more frequently and for longer periods, then they settle. In some they settle at once, but that is rare. In some they persist recurring till they are settled, that is less rare. In others the occurrence is at first at long intervals and waits for the consciousness to be ready.

*

It is quite right and part of the right consciousness in sadhana that you should feel drawn in your heart towards the Mother and aspire for the vision and realisation of her presence. But there should not be any kind of restlessness joined to this feeling. The feeling should be quietly intense. It will then be easier for the sense of the presence to come and grow in you.

*

Aspire to realisation, but do not be over-eager. Keep yourself quietly open and allow the Mother's force to work in you, that will bring the necessary realisation.

*

Things inside can be seen as distinctly as outward things whether in an image by the subtle vision or in their essence by a still more subtle and powerful way of seeing; but all these things have to develop in order to get their full power and intensity.

*

The sounds or voices you hear are like the sights (persons, objects) you see. As there is an inner sight other than the physical, so there is an inner hearing other than that of the external ear, and it can listen to voices and sounds and words of other worlds, other times and places, or those which come from supraphysical beings. But here you must be careful. If conflicting voices try to tell you what to do or not to do, you should not listen to them or reply. It is only myself and the Mother who can tell you what you should or should not do or guide or advise you.

*

Not only the experience of the higher but also the transformation of the lower nature is necessary. Pleasure, sadness, despair and sorrow are the ordinary play of the vital, impediments to progress — one has to go beyond them and bring down the vast unity and equality from above into the vital and in all the being.

Symbolic Meanings of Images & Objects

Aeroplane, Steamer, Train — Are always symbols of a rapid progress or forward movement.

Arrow — Is the symbol of the force which goes to its aim.

Ass — Is the symbol of the inertia and obstruction in the body.

Bird — Is the symbol of the individual soul.

Boar — Is rajasic strength and vehemence.

Book — Indicates some kind of knowledge.

Bow — Is a symbol of the force sent out to reach its mark.

Building — Is the symbol of a new creation.

Buffalo — Indicates rash and obscure vital force.

Bull — Is an emblem of strength and force.

Chakra — Chakras or circular movements are always the signs of energy in action, generally creative action.

Child (New Born) — Psychic Being.

Clouds — Are symbols of obscurity.

Conch — Is the call to realisation or the symbol of the spiritual call or the proclamation of victory.

Cow — In the Veda is the Divine Light.

Calf — Also is the Divine Light.

Cow (White) — Is the pure consciousness in which there is the Light.

Crane — Is the messenger of happiness.

Crown — Is the sign of fulfilment.

Dawn — Means an opening of some kind.

Deer — A symbol of speed in the spiritual progress.

Dog — Is the symbol of devoted affection and obedience.

Elephant — Is strength — sometimes strength illumined with wisdom.

Elephant-Golden — Strength of the true consciousness.

Fire — Symbolises tapasya, askesis or aspiration.

Fish — Is always the moving vital mind making all sorts of formations.

Flesh — A piece of flesh indicates something restless in the physical being.

FLOWERS — Indicate a blossoming in the consciousness.
FLUTE — Is the symbol of a call — usually the spiritual call.
FROG — Modest usefulness.
GOAT — Is often symbolic of lust.
HORSE — Is power — usually life-power, but also it may mean Mind-power or Tapas if it is dynamic and mobile.
INCENSE-STICKS — Adoration or consecration.
JUNGLE — Indicates unregenerated part of the vital nature.
LION — Indicates force and courage, and strength and power.
LOTUS — Is the symbol of the opening of the centres to the Light.
LOTUS (Red) — Sri Aurobindo's Consciousness.
LOTUS (White) — The Mother's Consciousness.
MILK — Is the knowledge and power descending from the Divine Consciousness.
MOON — Indicates spirituality.
MOUNTAIN — Represents the ascending planes of the higher consciousness towards the Divine.
PATAL — Simply means the subconscient below the Earth.
PEACOCK — Is the bird of victory.
PIGEON (White) — Peace.
PYRAMID — A symbol of aspiration.
RAIN — Descent of Grace or of the higher consciousness.
RIVER — Represents some movement of the consciousness of the vital plane.
ROSE (Golden) — Love and surrender full of the true consciousness.
ROSE (White) — Loving surrender to the Mother.
SEA — Indicates consciousness.
SERPENT (hooded) — Generally indicates future siddhi.
SERPENT (with 6 hoods) — Is the Kundalini Shakti.
SKY — Is a symbol of the mental consciousness (or the psychic).
SKY (Blue) — Higher Mind.
SNAKE — Indicates some kind of energy always — oftener bad, but it also can indicate some luminous or divine energy.
STAR — Signifies a creation or formation or the promise or power of a creation or formation.

SUDARSHAN-CHAKRA — Symbolises the action of Sri Krishna's force.
SUN — Is the symbol of the concentrated light of Truth.
SWAN — Is the symbol of the individual soul, the central being.
TOBACCO — Is associated with tamas.
TREE — Is the symbol of subconscient vital, spiritual life within.
VINA — Harmony.
WATER — Is the symbol of consciousness.

SYMBOLIC MEANINGS OF LIGHTS AND COLOURS

LIGHT — Indicates some kind of Force or Power.
LIGHT-BLUE — Is the fundamental colour of the Ananda.
DEEPER-BLUE — Is usually higher mind.
PALE-BLUE — Is illumined mind.
WHITISH-BLUE — Sri Krishna's Light.
LIGHT (White) — Is the Mother's Light, that of the Divine Consciousness in its essence.
SUN-LIGHT — Is the light of the Truth.
GOLDEN-LIGHT — Is the light of the Truth — the Supermind.
GOLDEN RED — Is the colour of the Supramental physical light, it has a strong transforming power.
GREEN (Light) — Is the vital energy or the life force. Light of emotion.
RED (Light) — Is the colour of the physical, when touched by the higher Light it becomes golden-red.
RED (Bright) — Divine Love or Force of the higher consciousness.
YELLOW LIGHT — Indicates Mind plane.
VIOLET — Is the light of Divine Grace and Compassion.
RAINBOW — Is the sign of peace and deliverance.

GENERAL TEACHINGS

All attachment is a hindrance to sadhana. Goodwill you should have for all, psychic kindness for all, but no vital attachment.

The love of the sadhak should be for the Divine. It is only when he has that fully that he can love others in the right way.

EIGHT CHAKRAS IN THE BODY:

The *Mūlādhāra* governs the physical down to the subconscient.

The abdominal centre — *Svādhiṣṭhāna* — governs the lower vital.

The navel centre — *Nābhipadma* or *Maṇipur* — governs the larger vital.

The heart centre — *Hṛdpadma* or *Anāhata* — governs the emotional being.

The throat centre — *Viśuddha* — governs the expressive and externalising mind.

The centre between the eye-brows — *Ājñācakra* — governs the dynamic mind, will, vision, mental formation.

The thousand-petalled lotus — *Sahasradala* — above, commands the higher thinking mind.

In our Yoga we mean by the *subconscient* that quite submerged part of our being in which there is no wakingly conscious and coherent thought, will or feeling or organised reaction, but which yet receives obscurely the impressions of all things and stores them up in itself and from it too all sort of stimuli, of persistent habitual movements, crudely repeated or disguised in strange forms can surge up into dream or into the waking nature.

Triple Universe: There is a vital plane above the *material* universe which we see; there is a *mental* plane above the vital and material. These three together — mental, vital, physical — are called the triple universe of the lower hemisphere.

Mind: The mind is a part of the nature which has to do with cognition and intelligence, with ideas, with mental or thought perceptions, the reactions of thought to things, with the truly mental movements and formations, mental vision and will etc. that are part of his intelligence.

Vital: The *vital* has to be carefully distinguished from mind, even though it has a mind element transfused into it; the vital is the Life nature made up of desires, sensations, feelings, passions, energies of action, will of desire, reactions of the desire soul in man and of all that play of possessive and other related instincts, anger, fear, greed, lust etc. that belong to this field of the nature.

Composition of man: The being of man is composed of these elements — the psychic being behind supporting all — the inner mental, vital and physical, and the outer, quite external nature of mind, life and body which is their instrument of expression. But above all is the central being (*Jīvātmā*) which uses them all for its manifestation: it is a portion of the Divine Self.

Central Being: The phrase 'central being' in our Yoga is usually applied to the portion of the Divine in us which supports all the rest and survives through death and birth. This central being has two forms — above, it is *Jīvātmā*, our true being, of which we become aware when the higher self-knowledge comes, — below, it is the *psychic being* which stands behind mind, body and life. The *Jīvātmā* is above the manifestation in life and presides over it; the psychic being stands behind the manifestation in life and supports it.

Purity means to accept no other influence but only the influence of the Divine.

Faithfulness means to admit and to manifest no other movements but only the movements prompted and guided by the Divine.

Sincerity means to lift all the movements of the being to the level of the highest consciousness and realisation already attained.

Sincerity exacts the unification and harmonisation of the whole being in all its parts and movements around the central Divine Will.

*

To deny in ignorance is no better than to affirm in ignorance.

*

In teaching Yoga to another one becomes to some extent a

master with disciples. The Yogis have always said that one who takes disciples, takes upon himself the difficulties of his disciples as well as one's own — that is why it is recommended not to take disciples unless and until one is siddha and even then only if one receives the Divine authority to do it. Secondly, there is the danger of egoism — when one is free from that, then the objection no longer holds.

*

If you want to be an instrument of the Truth, you must always speak the truth and not falsehood. But this does not mean that you must tell everything to everybody. To conceal the truth by silence or refusal to speak is permissible, because the truth may be misunderstood or misused by those who are not prepared for it or who are opposed to it — it may even be made a starting-point for distortion or sheer falsehood. But to speak falsehood is another matter. Even in jest it should be avoided, because it tends to lower the consciousness.

*

One who fears monotony and wants something new would not be able to do Yoga or at least this Yoga which needs an inexhaustible perseverance and patience.

*

The world will trouble you so long as any part of you belongs to the world. It is only if you belong entirely to the Divine that you can become free.

*

If you are not constant in aspiration, the nature will then sink back into the old lower ways.

*

This sadhana is not helped by fasting.

*

There is a future possibility of turning towards God for everyone, even for the atheist or the one who never thinks of God. The future possibility may only realise after ten thousand years and even then it can only come by practising Yoga.

*

The special Grace of the Divine is for the seekers of the Divine — for the others it is a Cosmic Will acting through their Karma.

*

That kind of Yogic Shakti is not the same as the Divine Shakti. Even the Asura and the Rakshasa have powers. The real Yoga Shakti is that which comes from contact or union with the Divine consciousness and its workings.

*

Spiritual aims and methods are not easy or natural (e.g., as quarrellings, sex-indulgence, greed, indolence, acquiescence in all imperfections are easy and natural) and if people become disciples, they are supposed to follow spiritual aims and endeavours, however hard and above ordinary nature and not the things that are easy and natural.

*

Allow a quiet and steady will to progress to be settled in you; learn the habit of a silent, persistent and thorough assimilation of what the Mother puts into you. This is the sound way to advance.

*

It is dangerous to think of giving up "all barriers of discrimination and defence against what is trying to descend" upon you. Have you thought what this would mean if what is descending is something not in consonance with the divine Truth, perhaps even adverse? An adverse Power would ask no better condition for getting control over the seeker. It is only the Mother's force and the Divine Truth that one should admit without barriers. And even there one must keep the power of discernment in order to detect anything false that comes masquerading as the Mother's force and the divine Truth, and keep too the power of rejection that will throw away all mixture.

If the central will is sincere, each recognition of a mistake can become a stepping-stone to a truer movement and a higher progress.

*

Remember the Mother and, though physically far from her, try to feel her with you and act according to what your inner being tells you would be her Will. Then you will be best able to feel her presence and mine and carry our atmosphere around you as a protection and a zone of quietude and light accompanying you everywhere.

*

The spiritual union must begin from within and spread out from there; it cannot be based on anything exterior — for, if so based, the union cannot be spiritual or real. That is the great mistake which so many make here: they put the whole emphasis on the external vital or physical relation with the Mother, insist on a vital interchange or else physical contact and when they do not get it to their satisfaction, enter into all kinds of disturbances, revolt, doubt, depression.

*

Even the physical must be able to feel invisibly the Mother's closeness, her concrete presence — then alone can the union be truly based and completed and then alone can any physical closeness or contact find its true value and fulfil its spiritual purpose. Till then any physical contact is value only so far as it helps the inner sadhana, but how much can be given and what will help or hinder, the Mother only can judge, the sadhak cannot be the judge.

*

The sadhaks always imagine in their ignorance that when the Mother sees more of one person than of another, it is because of personal preference and that she is giving more love and help to that person. That is altogether a mistake.

The only safe thing is to concentrate on the inner union foremost and altogether, to make that the one thing to be achieved and to leave aside all claims and demands for anything external, remaining satisfied with what the Mother gives and relying wholly on her wisdom and solicitude.

*

Those are the Mother's children closest to her who are open to her, close to her in her inner being, one with her will — not those who come bodily nearest to her.

*

To know the outer Mother truly one must know what is within

her and not look at the outer appearances only. That is only possible if one meets her with the inner being and grows into her consciousness — those who seek an outer relation only cannot do that.

*

If you keep the wideness and calm and also the love for the Mother in the heart, then all is safe — for it means the double foundation of the Yoga.

*

If they insist on seeing the Mother or on remaining when she wants them to go or are in a bad mood and throw it on her, it is very harmful for them to see her. Each should be contented with what the Mother gives them. The one thing important is to keep the inner attitude and establish the inner connection with the Mother independent of all outward circumstances.

*

Let the inner contact with the Mother increase — unless that is there, the outer contacts if too much multiplied easily degenerate into a routine.

*

But the coming near to the Mother should be in the inner rooms, not the outer. For in the inner rooms one can always enter and even arrange to stay there permanently.

*

Mistakes come from people bringing their ego, their personal feeling (likes and dislikes), their sense of prestige or their convenience, pride, sense of possession, etc. into the work. Harmony cannot be brought about by external organisation only; inner harmony there must be or else there will always be clash and disorder.

*

A contempt for others is out of place, especially since the Divine is in all. Evidently, the activities and aspirations of men are not trivial and worthless, for all life is a growth of the soul out of the darkness towards the Light. But our attitude is that humanity cannot grow out of its limitations by the ordinary means adopted by the human mind, politics, social reforms, philanthropy, etc. — these can only be temporary or local palliatives. The only true escape is a change of consciousness, a change into a greater, wider and purer way of being, and a life and action based upon that change.

*

The eye of the Yogin sees not only the outward events and persons and causes, but the enormous forces which precipitate them into action. When one is habituated to see the things behind, one is no longer prone to be touched by the outward aspects — or to expect any remedy from political, institutional or social changes; the only way out is through the descent of a consciousness which is not the puppet of these forces but is greater than they are and can force them either to change or disappear.

*

One must know that one is ignorant before one can begin to know.

*

When one feels the Divine and feels others in the Divine, then the real harmony comes. Meanwhile what there can be is the goodwill and unity founded on the feeling of a common divine goal and the sense of being all children of the Mother.

*

Each person has his own freedom of choice up to a certain point — unless he makes the full surrender. The Divine can lead, he does not drive. The help can only be offered, not imposed.

*

The Divine Grace is there ready to act at every moment, but it manifests as one grows out of the Law of Ignorance into the Law of Light.

*

One man who earnestly pursues the Yoga is of more value than a thousand well-known men.

*

The Yogi is one who is already established in realisation — the sadhak is one who is getting or still trying to get realisation.

*

Remember that no personality and no power is to be allowed to possess you. The Divine Force will not act in this way; it will work first to purify, to widen and enlighten the consciousness, to open it to Light and Truth, to awake the heart and the psychic being. Only afterwards will it take gradual and quiet control through a pure and conscious surrender.

*

Few are those from whom the Grace withdraws, but many are those who withdraw from the Grace.

*

It is not what others think of you that matters, but what you are yourself.

*

One rule for you I can lay down, "Do not do, say or think anything which you would want to conceal from the Mother".

*

Those who are able to open to the Divine receive Him — but also to those who can wait for the Divine, the Divine comes.

*

Cruelty and falsehood are the two things that separate most from the Divine.

*

He who would win high spiritual degrees, must pass endless tests and examinations. But most are anxious only to bribe the examiner.

*

Selfishness is the only sin, meanness the only vice, hatred the only criminality. All else can easily be turned into good, but these are obstinate resisters of deity.

*

The sign of dawning Knowledge is to feel that as yet I know

little or nothing; and yet, if I could only know my knowledge, I already possess everything.

*

Nothing in the world can be understood by itself, but only by that which is beyond it. If we would know all, we must turn our gaze to that which is beyond all.

*

Be cheerful and confident. Doubt and desire and Co. are there, no doubt, but the Divine is there also inside you. Open your eyes and look and look till the veil is rent and you see Him or Her.

*

When knowledge is fresh in us, then it is invincible; when it is old, it loses its virtue. This is because God moves always forward.

*

When people think of leaving the Ashram, it is not due to the pressure of Yoga, but to the pressure of something in them that negates the Yoga. If one follows one's psychic being and higher mental call, no amount of pressure of Yoga can produce such results. People talk as if the Yoga had some maleficent force in it which produces these results. It is on the contrary the resistance to Yoga that does it.

*

Beautiful is the face of the Divine Mother, but she too can be hard and terrible. Nay, then. is immortality a plaything to be given lightly to a child, or the divine life a prize without effort or the crown for a weakling? Strive rightly and thou shalt have; trust and thy trust shall in the end be justified; but the dread Law of the Way is there and none can abrogate it.

*

Those who are poor, ill-born and ill-bred are not the common herd; the common herd are all who are satisfied with pettiness and average humanity.

*

Rasa (taste) of poetry, painting or physical work is not the thing to go after. What gives the interest in Yoga is the *rasa* of the Divine and of the divine consciousness which means the *rasa* of Peace, of Silence, of inner Light and Bliss, of growing inner Knowledge, of increasing inner Power, of the Divine Love, of all the infinite fields of experience that open to one with the opening of the inner consciousness. The true *rasa* of poetry, painting or any other activity is only found when these things are part of the working of the Divine Force in you, and you feel it is that and it exists in the joy of that working.

*

Tobacco taken in any form spoils the spiritual atmosphere.

*

There is a sovereign royalty in taking no thought for oneself. To have needs is to assert a weakness; to claim something proves that we lack what we claim. To desire is to be impotent; it is to recognise our limitations and confess our incapacity to overcome them....

For all is within our reach, only the egoistic limits of our being prevents us from enjoying the whole universe as completely and concretely as we possess our own body and its immediate surroundings.

*

I have never said that this Yoga is a safe one — no Yoga is. Each has its dangers as has every great attempt in human life. But it can be carried through if one has a central sincerity and a fidelity to the Divine. These are the two necessary conditions.

The Mother:

As soon as you go deep enough, you meet something that is one in all. All meet in the Divine. But if you cannot feel one with somebody, it means you have not gone deep enough in your feeling.

*

As long as you remain in your corner and follow the course of the ordinary life, you are not touched or hurt; but once you come in contact with the Divine, there are only two ways open to you. You surrender and merge in it, and your surrender enlarges and glorifies you; or you revolt and all your possibilities are destroyed and your powers ebb away and are drawn from you into That which you oppose.

*

We find in others what is in us. If we always find mud around us it proves that there is mud somewhere in us.

*

Our best friend is he who loves us in the best of ourselves and yet does not ask us to be otherwise than we are.

*

Before deciding that something is wrong in others or in circumstances, you must be quite sure of the correctness of your judgment, — and which judgment is correct so long as one lives in the ordinary consciousness that is based on ignorance and filled with falsehood? Only the Truth-consciousness can judge. So it is better, in all circumstances, to leave the judgment to the Divine.

*

Titles give no value to a man unless he has acquired them in the service of the Divine.

*

Without the Divine life is a painful illusion, with the Divine all is bliss.... It is in a sincere consecration to the Divine that we can find relief from our too human sufferings.

*

The peace must be immense, the quietness deep and still, the calm unshakable, and the trust in the Divine ever-increasing.

*

The body should reject illness as energetically as in the mind we reject falsehood.

*

There are two methods of uniting oneself with the Divine. The one is to concentrate in the heart and go deep to find there His Presence; the other is to throw oneself into His arms, to nestle there, as a child nestles in the arms of its mother, with a complete surrender; and of these two the former seems to me to be easier.

*

From everybody is demanded only what he has, what he is, nothing more, but nothing less also.

*

If you are physically away from me and if you think of me all the time, you will be surely nearer to me than if you were seated near me but thinking about other things.

*

The best thing is to consider oneself neither great nor small, neither very important nor insignificant, because we are nothing by ourselves. We must want to be only what the Divine Will wants us to be.

*

The more one advances on the road the more modest one becomes and the more one sees that one has done nothing in comparison to what remains to be done. It is when one feels like a blind man that one begins to be ready for the illumination.

*

All fear must be overcome and replaced by a total confidence in the Divine Grace.

*

One cannot help others to overcome their griefs and sufferings unless one overcomes them in oneself and becomes master of one's sentiments and reactions.

*

It is not one person or the other that attracts you. It is the eternal feminine in the lower nature that attracts the eternal masculine in the lower nature and creates an illusion in the mind; it is the great play, obscure and half-conscious, of the forces of the unillumined Nature; and as soon as one succeeds in escaping from its blind and violent whirlpool, one perceives very soon that all desires and all attractions evaporate; there remains only the ardent aspiration towards the Divine.

*

Intellectual culture is indispensable for creating a good, wide, supple and rich mental instrument, but its action stops there.

For climbing above the mind it is more often a hindrance than a help, because, in general, a refined and educated mind finds its satisfaction in itself and rarely wants to remain silent for being surpassed.

*

I have always thought that something in the character of the teacher was responsible for the indiscipline of his students. It is not with severity but with self-control that one can govern the children.

*

To will what God wills — that is the supreme secret.

*

To the Divine you are worth no more than what you have given Him.

*

Let us be always very careful to avoid all that might encourage in us the spirit of display.

*

A noblest courage is to recognise one's faults.

*

To be above offence or insult makes one truly great.

*

To speak always the truth is the highest title of nobility.

*

It is through Beauty that the Divine manifests in the physical, in the mental through Knowledge, in the vital through Power, and in the psychic through Love.

*

An impulsive person who cannot control himself has a disordered life. Do not act under an impulse.

*

The nobility of a being is measured by its capacity of gratitude.

*

Concentration upon oneself means decay and death — concentration on the Divine alone brings life and growth and realisation.

*

Closeness to the Divine will always grow with the growth of consciousness, equanimity and love.

*

Jealousy comes from a narrowness of the mind and a weakness of the heart. It is a great pity that so many are attacked by it.

*

A very very quiet head is indispensable for a clear understanding and vision and a right action.

*

Do not mind the stupidity of others, mind yours.

*

All the lower movements have to be conquered if ever anything divine is to be established upon earth.

*

Each one is given what he truly needs, in fact what he is capable of receiving and utilising. If he asks for more I rarely refuse to give — but often it is more than what he can receive and then it creates a disorder and sometimes even a catastrophe.

*

It is the Divine Presence that gives value to life. This Presence is the source of all peace, all joy, all security. Find this Presence in yourself and all your difficulties will disappear.

*

When you give yourself to the accomplishment of an unselfish aim, never expect the ordinary people to praise and support you. On the contrary they will always fight against you, hate and curse you. But the Divine will be with you.

*

It is a dangerous illness: laziness.

*

I am always seated in your heart, consciously living in you.

*

In order to progress, Nature destroys while the Divine Consciousness stimulates growth and finally transforms.

*

To recognise the presence of a "disharmonious atmosphere" is useful only so far as it makes in each one the will to change it into a harmonious atmosphere and to do that the first important step is for each one to get out of his own limited point of view in order to understand the point of view of others. It is more important for each one to find the mistake in himself rather than insist on the mistake of others.

*

Do not forget even for a moment that all this has been created by Him out of Himself. Not only He is present in everything, but also He is everything. The differences are only in expression and manifestation. If you forget this you lose everything.

*

If you refuse to become a docile and surrendered servant of the Divine and of the Master who manifests Him, it means that you will remain a slave of your egoism, your vanity, your presumptuous ambition, and a toy in the hands of the Rakshasas who allure you with brilliant images in their attempt — not always unsuccessful — to possess you.

*

One must be able to control oneself before one can hope to govern others.

*

Always circumstances come to reveal the hidden weaknesses that have to be overcome.

*

When temptation comes, resist it — do not yield to it.

*

By yogic discipline one can not only foresee destiny but can alter it, change it almost wholly.

*

If you obey all your fancies, you will never get control over yourself, it is your fancies that will control you. Most people when they feel bored, instead of making an endeavour to rise one step higher in their consciousness, come down one step lower; they come down even below the level where they were and they do most stupid things. They make themselves vulgar in the hope of amusing themselves. That is how men take to drink, spoil their health, deaden their brain. If they had risen instead of falling they would have profited by the occasion in making a progress.

In calamities, when it is very painful, they seek what they call "diversion", they do stupid things, drag their consciousness down, instead of raising it. If there is anything extremely painful happening to you, never try to deaden yourself, to forget, to descend into unconsciousness. Rather to go forward, get into the heart of your grief: you will find there the light, the truth, the force and the joy which the pain hides. But for that you must be firm and refuse to slip down.

*

Honesty is indispensable for Yoga.

To try to cheat the Divine is worse than to try to cheat a human being and much more foolish.

*

The true power is always quiet. Restlessness, agitation, impatience are the sure signs of weakness and imperfection.

*

The closer you come to the Divine, the more you live under a shower of overwhelming evidence of His immeasurable Grace.

*

The true consciousness is incapable of feeling superior. It is only the small consciousness that seeks to show superiority. Even a child is more developed than such a being; for it is spontaneous in its movements. Rise above all smallness. Do not be interested in any other thing than your relation with the Divine, what you wish to do for Him.

GODS

The Gods, as has already been said, are in origin and essence permanent Emanations of the Divine put forth from the Supreme by the Transcendent Mother, the Adya Shakti.

The Adya Shakti is the Supreme Consciousness and Power above the universe and it is by her that all the Gods are manifested, and even the Supramental Ishwara comes into manifestation through her.

The Gods cannot be transformed, for they are typal and not evolutionary beings, they can come for conversion, that is to say, to give up their own ideas and outlook on things and conform themselves to the higher Will and Supramental Truth of the Divine.

There is and can be no psychic being in a non-evolutionary creature like the Asura; there can be none in a god who does not need one for his existence. But what the god has is a Purusha and a Prakriti or Energy of nature of that Purusha. If any being of the typal worlds wants to evolve, he has to come down to earth and take a human body and accept to share in the evolution.

*

There is only one psychic being for each human being, but the beings of the higher planes e.g., the Gods of the Overmind can manifest in more than one human body at a time by sending different emanations into different bodies.

*

The Overmind is the world of the gods and the gods are not merely powers but have forms also. It is the physical mind which believes only what is physical that denies them.

*

Whatever name is called the Power that answers is the Mother. Each name indicates a certain aspect of the Divine and is limited by that aspect; the Mother's Power is universal.

The Mother:

Sri Aurobindo ... speaks of the gods of the Overmind who are very much like human beings; they are infinitely greater and more powerful, but with characteristics and reactions very similar to those of men. Beyond them one experiences the impersonal Divine. But beyond this experience is the Divine who is the Person himself. To reach this transcendent supreme Person (*Puruṣottama*) one has to pass through the impersonal.

Symbolic Meanings of Gods

Adya Shakti — Is the original Shakti, therefore, the highest form of the Mother.

Brahma, Vishnu, Shiva — Are only three powers and personalities of the one Cosmic Godhead.

Brahma — Is the power of the Divine that stands behind formation and creation.

Vishnu — Being the creator, all the three gods are often spoken of as creating the universe — even Shiva who is by tradition the Destroyer.

Shiva — is the Lord of Tapas. The Power is the power of Tapas.

Devi — Is the Divine Shakti — the Consciousness and Power of the Divine, the Mother and Energy of the worlds.

Durga — The lion with Durga on it is the symbol of the Divine

Consciousness acting through a divinised physical-vital and Vital-emotional force.

KALI AND MAHAKALI — Are not the same. Kali is a lesser form. Mahakali in the higher planes appears usually with golden colour.

GODS — Are the powers that stand above the world and transmit the divine workings.

GANESH — Is the power that removes obstacles by the force of Knowledge. He is a god of spiritual Knowledge.

HANUMAN — Perfect Bhakti.

KARTIKEYA — Represents victory over the hostile powers. He is also the leader of the divine forces.

SRI KRISHNA — Is the Lord of divine love and ananda — and his flute calls the physical being to awake out of the attachments of the physical world and turn to that love and ananda.

RADHA — Is the personification of the absolute love for the Divine, total and integral in all parts of the being from the highest spiritual to the physical, bringing the absolute self-giving and total consecration of all the being and calling down into the body and the most material nature the supreme Ananda.

GREAT MEN

People have begun to try to prove that great men were not great, which is a very big mistake. If greatness is not appreciated by men, the world will become mean, small, dull, narrow and tamasic.

*

Outer greatness is not the aim of Yoga. But that is no reason why one should not recognise the part played by greatness in the order of the universe or the place of great men of action, great poets and artists, etc. It is the power in them that is great and that power comes from the Divine — by their actions and greatness they help the world and aid the cosmic purpose.

*

Vices are simply an overflow of energy in irregulated channels. Great men have more energy and the energy comes out in what men call vices as well as in what men call virtues. Why should the Divine care for the vices of great men? Is he a policeman? So long as one is in the ordinary nature, one has capacities and defects, virtues and vices. When one goes beyond, there are no virtues and vices, — for these things do not belong to the Divine Nature.

*

There are some men who are self-evidently superhuman, great spirits who are only using the human body. Europe calls them supermen, we call them Vibhutis. They are manifestations of Nature, of divine power presided over by a spirit commissioned for the purpose, and that spirit is an emanation from the Almighty, who accepts human strength and weakness but is not bound by them. They are above morality and ordinarily without a conscience, acting according to their own nature. For they are not men developing upwards from the animal to the divine and struggling against their lower natures, but beings already fulfilled and satisfied with themselves. Even the holiest of them have a contempt for the ordinary law and custom and break them easily and without remorse.

*

The Rakshasa is the supreme and thoroughgoing individualist, who believes life to be meant for his own untrammelled self-fulfilment and self-assertion. A necessary element in humanity, he is particularly useful in revolutions. The Rakshasa is not an altruist. If by satisfying himself he can satisfy others, he is pleased; but he does not make that his motive. If he has to trample on others to satisfy himself, he does so without compunction. The Rakshasa has Kama, he has no Prema. But the Vibhuti, though he takes self-gratification and enjoyment on his way, never comes for self-gratification and enjoyment. He comes, for work, to help man on his way, the world in its evolution.

HUMAN PROGRESS

Inferior mankind gravitates downward from mind towards life and body; average mankind dwells constantly in mind limited by and looking towards life and body; superior mankind levitates upward either to idealised mentality or to pure idea, direct truth of knowledge and spontaneous truth of existence; supreme mankind rises to divine beatitude and from that level either goes upward to pure Sat and Parabrahman or remains to beatify its lower members and raise to divinity in itself and others — this human existence.

HUMAN SERVICE

All work done in an egoistic spirit, however good for people in the world of Ignorance, is of no avail to the seeker of the Yoga.

*

The idea of usefulness to humanity is the old confusion due to secondhand ideas imported from the West. Obviously, to be 'useful' to humanity there is no need of Yoga; everyone who leads the human life is useful to humanity in one way or another.

Yoga is directed towards God, not towards man. If a divine supramental consciousness and power can be brought down and established in the material world, that obviously would mean an immense change for the earth including humanity and its life.

But the effect on humanity would only be one result of the change; it cannot be the object of the sadhana. The object of the sadhana can only be to live in the divine consciousness and to manifest it in life.

*

To concentrate most on one's own spiritual growth and experience is the first necessity of the sadhak — to be eager to help others draws away from the inner work. To grow in the spirit is the greatest help one can give to others, for then something flows out naturally to those around that helps them.

*

Working for family, society, country is a larger ego — it is not the Divine. One can work for them and say that one is working for the Divine only if one is conscious of the Divine Adesh to act for that purpose or of the Divine Force working within him. Otherwise it is only an idea of the mind identifying country etc. with the Divine.

*

The attainment of God is the true object of all human effort for which all the other efforts political, social, literary, intellectual, are only a necessary condition and preparation of the race; but there are both differences in the state of the attainment, differences in its range and effectivity.

*

Selfishness kills the soul; destroy it. But take care that your altruism does not kill the souls of others. Very usually, altruism is only the sublimest form of selfishness.

*

Do not be caught by the desire to "help" others — do and speak yourself the right thing from the inner poise and leave the help to come to them from the Divine. Nobody can really help — only the Divine Grace.

Altruism, philanthropy, the service of mankind are in themselves mental or moral ideals, not laws of the spiritual life.... The greatest service to humanity, the surest foundation for its true progress, happiness and perfection is to prepare or find the way by which the individual and the collective man can transcend the ego and live in its true self, no longer bound to ignorance, incapacity, disharmony and sorrow.

*

This erring race of human beings dreams always of perfecting their environment by the machinery of Government and society; but it is only by the perfection of the soul within that the outer environment can be perfected. What thou art within, that outside thee thou shalt enjoy; no machinery can rescue thee from the law of thy being.

The Mother:

Yoga is not for the sake of humanity but for the sake of Divinity. It is not the welfare of humanity that we seek but the manifestation of the Divine. We are here to work out the Divine Will so that we may be its instruments for the progressive incorporation of the Supreme and the establishment of His reign upon earth. Only that portion of humanity which will respond to the Divine Call shall receive its Grace.

*

One of the commonest forms of ambition is the idea of service to humanity. All attachment to such service or work is a sign of personal ambition. There should be no attachment to any objcet or any mode of life. You must be absolutely free.

*

It is an illusion to think that all these so-called movements change things. It is merely taking a cup and beating the water in it. This illusion of action is one of the greatest illusions of human nature. Men have a feeling that if they are not all the time running about and bursting into fits of feverish activity, they are doing nothing. Whatever has been done in the world has been done by the very few who can stand outside the action in silence; for it is they who are the instruments of the Divine Power. They are dynamic agents, conscious instruments; they bring down the forces that change the world. Things can be done in that way, not by a restless activity. In peace, in silence and in quietness the world was built; and each time that something is to be truly built, it is in peace and silence and quietness that it must be done. I am not speaking of the ordinary day-to-day acts that are needed for the common external life, but of those who have or believe that they have something to do for the world. Enter into the consciousness of Eternity, then only you will know what true action is.

*

Change yourself if you wish to change the world. Let your inner transformation be the proof that a truth-consciousness can take possession of the material world and that the Divine's Unity can be manifested upon earth.

*

Organisations, however vast and complex they may be, can achieve nothing permanent, unless a new force, more divine and all-powerful, expresses itself through a perfected human instrument.

*

The conditions under which men live upon earth are the result of their state of consciousness. To seek to change the conditions without changing the consciousness is a vain chimera; for no human organisation can change radically unless human consciousness itself changes.

*

In this effort, however, to improve human conditions there have always been two tendencies, which although apparently contrary to each other should rather be complementary and together work out the progress. One seeks a collective reorganisation, something that would lead towards an effective unity of mankind: the other declares that all progress is made first by the individual and insists that it is the individual who should be given conditions in which he can progress freely. Both are equally true and necessary, and our effort should be directed along both the lines.

All urge of rivalry, all struggle for precedence and domination, should disappear giving place to a will for harmonious organisation, for clear-sighted and effective collaboration.

For all world organisation, to be real and to be able to live, must be based upon mutual respect and understanding between nation and nation as well as between individual and individual. It is only in the collective order and organisation, in a collaboration based upon mutual goodwill that lies the possibility of man being lifted out of the painful chaos where he is now.

This must not be understood, however, to mean that each nation would choose its place arbitrarily, through its ambition and its greed. A country's mission is not a thing to be settled mentally, with all the egoistic and ignorant preferences of the external consciousness; that would serve only to shift the field of the conflict between nations, but the conflict would continue, perhaps more accentuated.

*

For those who practise the integral Yoga, the welfare of humanity can be only a consequence and a result, it cannot be the aim. ...So we can say that on the one hand a change in the human consciousness is absolutely indispensable; on the other hand, without an integral transformation of the terrestrial atmosphere, the conditions of human life cannot be effectively changed. The appearance of a new force and light and power, accompanying the descent of the supramental consciousness into this world can alone lift man out of the agony and pain and misery under which he is submerged. The integral Yoga is not an escape from the physical world leaving it irrevocably to its fate. Nor is it an acceptance of the material life as it is with no hope for any decisive change, an acceptance of the world as the final expression of the Divine Will. It is only the possession of the consciousness of the divine nature in its essence that enables one to have the conception of what the divine nature will be in its manifestation. Yet they who have realised in themselves this consciousness are generally more anxious to become the superman than to give a description of it.

*

No material organisation, whatever its degree of preparation, is capable of bringing a solution to the miseries of man.

Man must rise to a higher level of consciousness and get rid of his ignorance, limitation and selfishness in order to get rid also of his sufferings.

HUMAN UNITY

It is not by social and political devices, or at any rate not by these, chiefly or only, that the unity of the human race can be enduringly or fruitfully accomplished....

Nature moves forward always in the midst of all stumblings and secures her aims in the end more often in spite of man's imperfect mentality than by its means....

Man must learn not to suppress and mutilate, but to fulfil himself in the fulfilment of mankind, even as he must learn not to mutilate or destroy, but to complete his ego by expanding it out of its limitations and losing it in something greater....

A national culture, a national religion, a national education may be useful things provided they do not interfere with the growth of human solidarity on the one side and individual freedom of thought and conscience and development on the other; for they give form to the communal soul and help it to add its quota to the sum of human advancement; but a State education, a State religion, a State culture are unnatural violences....

Human society progresses really and vitally in proportion as law becomes the child of freedom; it will reach its perfection when, man having learned to know and become spiritually one with his fellow-men, the spontaneous law of his society exists only as the outward mould of his self-governed inner liberty....

The first principle of human unity, groupings being necessary, should be a system of free and natural groupings which would leave no room for internal discords, incompatibilities and repression and revolt as between race and race or people and people....

The union of liberty and equality can only be achieved by the power of human brotherhood and it cannot be founded on anything else. But brotherhood exists only in the soul and by the soul; it can exist by nothing else. For this brotherhood is not a matter either of physical kinship or of vital association or of intellectual agreement. When the soul claims freedom, it is the freedom of its self-development of the divine in man in all his being. When it claims equality, what it is claiming is that freedom equally for all and the recognition of the same soul, the same godhead in all human beings. When it strives for brotherhood, it is founding that equal freedom of self-development on a common aim, a common life, a unity of mind and feeling founded upon the recognition of this inner spiritual unity. These three things are in fact the nature of the soul; for freedom, equality, unity are the eternal attributes of the Spirit. It is the practical recognition of this truth, it is the awakening of the soul in man and the attempt to get him to live from his soul and not from his ego which is the inner meaning of religion, and it is that to which the religion of humanity also must arrive before it can fulfil itself in the life of the race....

*

This is the cause why all human systems have failed in the end; for they have never been anything but a partial and confused application of reason to life.... For the limited imperfect human reason has no self-sufficient light of its own; it is obliged to proceed by observation, by experiment, by action, through errors and stumblings to a larger experience.

*

There has been almost continuous war in the world. Man is a quarrelling and fighting animal and so long as he is so how can there be peace?

The Mother:

It is only by the growth and establishment of the consciousness of human unity, that a true and lasting peace can be achieved upon earth. All means leading towards this goal are welcome, although the external ones have a very limited effect; however, the most important, urgent and indispensable of all is a transformation of the human consciousness itself, an enlightenment of and conversion in its working....

*

If diplomacy could become the instrument of the Truth and the Divine Grace, instead of being based on duplicity and falsehood, a big step would be taken towards human unity and harmony.

IGNORANCE (MAYA)

Ignorance means Avidya, the seperative consciousness and the egoistic mind and life that flow from it and all that is natural to the separative consciousness and the egoistic mind and life. This Ignorance is the result of a movement by which the cosmic intelligence separated itself from the light of the Supermind and lost the Truth. It is this that some of the ancient thinkers like Shankara, not perceiving the greater Truth-Force behind, stigmatised as Maya and thought to be the highest creative power of the Divine.

Falsehood, on the other hand, is not this Avidya, but an extreme result of it. It is created by an Asuric power which intervenes in this creation and is not only separated from the Truth and therefore limited in knowledge and open to error, but in revolt against the Truth, or in the habit of seizing the Truth only to pervert it.

*

I have started writing about doubt, but even in doing so I am afflicted by the 'doubt' whether any amount of writing or of anything else can ever persuade the eternal doubt in man which is the penalty of his native ignorance. For doubt exists for its own sake; its very function is to doubt always and, even when convinced, to go on doubting still; it is only to persuade its entertainer to give it board and lodging that it pretends to be an honest truth-seeker.

*

Nothing can arise from Nothing. Asat, Maya, nothingness, is a creation of our mind. Out of its own incapacity it has created the conception of a zero; but it is an incalculable Infinite. Our sense by its incapacity has invented darkness. In truth there is nothing but Light. God is everywhere and wherever God is, there is Light.

*

There is no way to get free from ignorance and ego except to open to the higher consciousness so that it may descend and open to the Mother.

*

The difficulty of the difficulties is self-created, a knot of the Ignorance; when a certain inner perception loosens the knot, the worst of the difficulty is over.

The Mother:

The more a mind is ignorant the more easily it judges everything it does not know or is incapable of understanding.

ILLNESS

Illness marks some imperfection or weakness or else opening to adverse touches in the physical nature and is often connected also with some obscurity or disharmony in the lower vital or the physical mind or elsewhere.

It is very good if one can get rid of illness entirely by faith and Yoga-power or the influx of the Divine Force. But very often this is not altogether possible, because the whole nature is not open or able to respond to the Force.

*

Attacks of illness are attacks of the lower nature or of adverse forces taking advantage of some weakness, opening or response in the nature — like all other things that come and they have got to be thrown away, they come from outside.

Certainly, one can act from within on an illness and cure it. Only it is not always easy as there is much resistance in Matter, a resistance of inertia. An untiring persistence is necessary.

If you can succeed by the inner action in preventing increase, even that is something; you have then by practice to strengthen the power till it becomes able to cure. Note that so long as the power is not entirely there, some aid of physical means need not be altogether rejected.

All illnesses pass through the nervous or vital-physical sheath of the subtle consciousness and subtle body before they enter the physical. If one is conscious of the subtle body or with the subtle consciousness, one can stop an illness on its way and prevent it from entering the physical body.

*

It is only by the conquest of the material nature that illness can cease altogether to come.

In illness physical means can be used wherever necessary; but behind the physical means there must be the Divine Force. The physical means are to be used with discrimination and in case of necessity.

*

The human body has always been in the habit of answering to whatever forces chose to lay hands on it and illness is the price it pays for its inertia and ignorance. It has to learn to answer to the one Force alone, but that is not easy for it to learn.

*

All these ideas are wrong suggestions to which you must refuse access. You have the Mother's Grace and presence with you and it is only when you allow such suggestions of restlessness and despair that this kind of condition is created. Otherwise when you receive the Force it works. However serious an attack may be or however severe the illness, it can be got rid of by receptivity to the true working. If that is not enough, the Force aided by treatment can deal with them. The worst possible diseases have been cured recently by the Mother's force aided by treatment and this in people who know nothing of sadhana. In a sadhak the action can be still more effective. But the first thing is to get rid of these dark and disabling suggestions and open yourself once more to the Mother's working.

The Mother:

All the time he is busy with that idea and he has made a strong formation of illness around him. He is unable to receive my help because of this formation. Let him discard the idea of illness and more than half the trouble will be over and it will be easy to cure him.

*

If you want to get cured from illness there are two conditions. First you must be without fear, absolutely fearless and secondly you must have a complete faith in the Divine Protection. These two things are essential.

Modern medicine lays a great stress on microbic infection and the dictum is to kill the microbes and the disease will be cured and it is so in many cases, but for us, illness has other deeper causes. It is an expression of a disorder of an inner subtler kind. If you cannot reach and touch that you cannot be free from illness or prevent it from recurring....

Illness always, without exception, means a disturbance of equilibrium.... Now with regard to the causes, they are innumerable: there are inner or personal causes and there are external causes....

To resist the attack of illness, you must become fighters of the vital, spiritual fighters in your vital. All who do Yoga sincerely must become so, and when they can become they are quite safe. But one of the conditions enabling you to become such a fighter is that you must never have an evil will or an evil thought against anyone. For if you have a bad feeling or a bad will or a bad thought against people, you at once bring yourself down to their level and then you receive their blows.

The first thing to do then is to quiet oneself, to bring the peace and calm, the repose and a full confidence not necessarily, into the entire body, but into the affected part. And then you can see the cause of the disorder. Even if you cannot in the beginning spot the central cause, you can try to get something near to it, approximating to it. And then you throw the light of consciousness, the spiritual force, exerting a kind of pressure upon the source of the disturbance and you try to re-establish balance and normal functioning of the affected part.

Now, there are, much nearer, in the physical, in the terrestrial atmosphere a large number of small beings whom you do not see, because your sight is too limited, but who move about in your atmosphere. There are some who are very good and nice, others who are wicked. Mostly these entities are the offshoots of the disintegration of vital beings, of persons who have died and are on the way of gradual dissolution. Often they are seized by Asuric forces and used by them as their instruments for all kinds of mischief.... Very often they are behind accidents that happen to people. They get immense pleasure in the disorder and confusion following an accident. It not only amuses them but gives them their food. They draw sustenance from the human vitality thrown out of the body by emotion and excitement and all that. And further, these beings are not harmonious among themselves. They quarrel, they fight, they dash against each other, want to hit and destroy one another. And this is the origin of microbes. Microbes are forces of disintegration, the living remnants, scattered bits of the vital passions and desires and hungers of dead people, taken possession of by the vital beings, asuric beings. Most of the microbes have behind them a bad will and this is what makes them so dangerous. Unless one knows the quality and the kind of the bad will behind and can act upon it, in 99 cases out of 100, one is unable to find the true and the total remedy. The microbe is only the most material expression of some entity which is living, the embodiment in the most physical of a vital force....

Now when it is a case of attack from adverse forces, the thing becomes still more and specially complex.... There is a force outside you that wants to do you harm. You must have opened the door by a spiritual error of yours: a movement of vanity, anger, spite, violence; it may be even a momentary lapse and that is sufficient to give an opportunity to the beings that are always there on the watch for it.... Then the first method I spoke of is not sufficient. You have to add to it another aid, you must add the force of spiritual purification. It is such an absolutely and perfectly constructive force that no destructive force can stand before it.... The adverse force usually disappears forthwith, for if it falls within the range of the force of light it gets dissolved. No force of disintegration can face this force of purifying fire and light. Either it is reduced to nothing or it has to change into a force of construction. In either case you are not only freed of your illness, but all possibility of its return is eliminated.

That does not necessarily mean that one is safe from all possible attack. To say the truth, — it is only when one has permanently established his consciousness in the supramental that the body is protected from all adverse attacks and inner disharmony.

ADVICE TO A SICK DISCIPLE:

You must not fear. Most of your troubles come from fear. In fact, 90 per cent of illnesses are the result of the subconscient fear in the body. In the ordinary consciousness of the body there is a more or less hidden anxiety about the consequences of the slightest physical disturbance. It can be translated by these words of doubt about the future: "And what will happen?". It is this anxiety that must be checked. Indeed this anxiety is a lack of confidence in the Divine's Grace, the unmistakable sign that the consecration is not complete and perfect.

As a practial means of overcoming this subconscient fear each time that something of it comes at the surface, the more enlightened part of the being must impress on the body the necessity of an entire trust in the Divine's Grace, the certitude that this Grace is always working for the best in ourself as well as in all, and the determination to submit entirely and unreservedly to the Divine's Will.

The body must know and be convinced that its essence is divine and that if no obstacle is put in the way of the Divine's working nothing can harm us. This process must be steadily repeated until all recurrence of fear is stopped. And then even if the illness succeeds in making its appearance, its strength and duration will be considerably diminished until it is definitively conquered.

IMMORTALITY

Immortality is one of the possible results of supramentalisation, but it is not an obligatory result and it does not mean that there will be an eternal or indefinite prolongation of life as it is. To live in the Divine and have the Divine Consciousness is itself immortality and to be able to divinise the body also and make it a fit instrument for divine works and divine life would be its material expression only.

There can be no immortality of the body without supramentalisation; the potentiality is there in the Yogic force and Yogis can live for 200 or 300 years or more, but there can be no real principle of it without the Supramental.

INTELLECT

It is not by the intellect that one can progress in the Yoga but by psychic and spiritual receptivity — as for knowledge and true understanding, it grows in sadhana by the growth of the intuition, not of the physical intellect.

That is why one has to object to the intellect thrusting itself in as the all-knowing judge; if it kept to its own limits, there would be no objection to it. But it makes constructions of words and ideas which have no application to the Truth, babbles foolish things in its ignorance and makes its constructions a wall which refuses to let in the Truth that surpasses its own capacities and scope.

*

The psychic being will not need the support of intellectual ideas or outer signs and helps. It is that alone that can give you the direct feeling of the Divine, the constant nearness, the inner support and aid. You will not then feel the Mother remote or have any further doubt about the realisation; for the mind thinks and the vital craves, but the soul feels and knows the Divine.

*

To see the Truth does not depend on a big intellect or a small intellect. It depends on being in contact with the Truth and the mind silent and quiet to receive it. The biggest intellects can make errors of the worst kind and confuse Truth and Falsehood, if they have not the contact with the Truth or the direct experience.

*

The point is that people take no trouble to see whether their intellect is giving them right thoughts, right conclusions, right views on things and persons, right indications about their conduct or course of action. They have their idea and accept it as truth or follow it simply because it is their idea. Even when they recognise that they have made mistakes of the mind, they do not consider it of any importance nor do they try to be more careful mentally than before. The intellect, it is said, is man's highest instrument and he must think and act according to its ideas. But this is not true; the intellect needs an inner light to guide, check and control it quite as much as the vital. There is something above the intellect which one has to discover and the intellect should be only an intermediary for the action of that source of true Knowledge.

*

But for many intellectuals, so called, their intellectuality may be a stumbling-block as they bind themselves with mental conceptions or stifle their psychic fire under the heavy weight of rational thought.

*

Yoga is not a field for intellectual argument or dissertation. It is not by the exercise of the logical or the debating mind that one can arrive at a true understanding of Yoga or follow it. Unless and until the mind is stilled, including the intellectual or logical mind, and opens itself in quietude or silence to a higher and deeper consciousness, vision and knowledge, sadhana cannot reach its goal. For the same reason an unquestioning openness to the Guru is demanded in the Indian spiritual tradition.

*

Out of one thousand mental questions and answers there are only one or two here and there that are really of any dynamic assistance — while a single inner response or a little growth of consciousness will do what those thousand questions and answers could not do.

*

What I write usually helps only the mind and that too very little, for people do not really understand what I write — they put their own constructions on it. People do not understand what I write because the mind by itself cannot understand things that are beyond it.

*

For one who wants to practise sadhana, sadhana must come first — reading and mental development can only be subordinate things. Mental development may or may not help sadhana — if the mind is too intellectually developed in certain rationalistic lines, it may hinder.

*

It is impossible for the limited human reason to judge the way or purpose of the Divine, — which is the way of the Infinite dealing with the finite.

*

So long as we confine ourselves to sense-evidence and the physical consciousness, we can conceive nothing and know nothing except the material world and its phenomena.

*

For training the intellect you should look at things without egoism or prejudice or haste, to try to know fully and accurately before judging, to try to see the truth behind other opinions than your own etc., etc.

*

The intellect can be as great an obstacle as the vital when it chooses to prefer its own constructions to the Truth.

*

The knowledge of God is not to be gained by weighing the feeble arguments of reason for or against His existence; it is to be gained only by a self-transcending and absolute consecration, aspiration and experience.

*

Man's road to spiritual supermanhood will be open when he declares boldly that all he has yet developed, including the intellect of which he is so rightly and yet so vainly proud, are now no longer sufficient for him, and that to uncase, discover, set free this greater Light within shall be henceforward his pervading preoccupation.

The Mother:

Whether the intellect is a help or a hindrance depends upon the person and upon the way in which it is used. There is a true movement of the intellect and there is a wrong movement; one helps, the other hinders. The intellect that believes too much in its importance and wants satisfaction for its own sake, is an obstacle to the higher realisation. A power has the right movement when it is set into activity for the Divine purpose; it has the wrong movement when it is set into activity for its own satisfaction.

INTERMEDIATE ZONE

Any one passing the border of ordinary consciousness can enter into this intermediate zone of vital world, if he does not take care to enter into the psychic. In itself there is no harm in passing through, provided one does not stop there. But ego, sex, ambition, etc. if they get exaggerated, can easily lead to a dangerous downfall ... or there is the opposite danger that he may become the instrument of some apparently brilliant but ignorant formation; for these intermediate planes are full of little Gods or strong Daityas or smaller beings who want to create, to materialise something or to enforce a mental and vital formation in the earth life and are eager to use or influence or even possess the thought and will of the sadhak and make him their instrument for the purpose. This is quite apart from the well-known danger of actually hostile beings whose sole purpose is to create confusion, falsehood corruption of the sadhana and disastrous unspiritual error.

*

The main strength of the hostile forces is in the vital — but there are some in the lower ranges of mind and smaller beings and forces in the subtle physical also.

KARMA

Karma is only a machinery, it is not the fundamental cause of terrestrial existence — it cannot be, for when the soul first entered this existence, it had no Karma.

*

If we believe that the soul is repeatedly reborn in the body, we must believe also that there is some link between the lives that preceded and the lives that follow and that the past of the soul has an effect on its future; and that is the spiritual essence of the law of Karma.

The idea of reward or retribution is a crude and vulgar conception which is a mere popular error.

*

We must leave far behind us the current theory of Karma and its shallow attempt to justify the ways of the Cosmic Spirit by forcing on them a crude identity with the summary notions of law and justice, the crude and often savagely primitive methods of reward and punishment, lure and deterrent dear to the surface human mind. There is here a more authentic and spiritual truth at the base of Nature's action and a far less mechanically calculable movement. Here is no rigid and narrow ethical law bound down to a petty human significance, no teaching of a child soul by a mixed system of blows and lollipops, no unprofitable wheel of a brutal cosmic justice automaticlly moved in the traces of man's ignorant judgments and earthly desires and instincts. Life and rebirth do not follow these artificial constructions, but a movement spiritual and intimate to the deepest intention of Nature....

Its complexities cannot be unravelled by our physical mind ever bound up in the superficial appearance, nor by our vital mind of desire stumbling forward in the cloud of its own instincts and longings and rash determinations through the maze of these myriad favouring and opposing forces that surround and urge and drive and hamper us from the visible and invisible worlds. Nor can it be perfectly classified, accounted for, tied up in bundles by the precisions of our logical intelligence in its inveterate search for clear-cut dogmas. On that day only shall we perfectly decipher what is now to us Nature's obscure hieroglyph of Karma when there rises in our enlarged consciousness the supramental way of knowledge.

The Mother:

On the highest height is the Supreme and in the lowest depth is matter; and there is an infinite gradation of levels of consciousness between this lowest depth and the highest height. In the plane of matter and on the level of the ordinary consciousness you are bound hand and foot. A slave to the mechanism of Nature, you are tied to the chain of Karma. There is an illusion of independent movement, but in fact you repeat what all others do. But it need not be so. You can shift your place if you will. You can rise and look from above and by changing your consciousness you can even change the consequences. This precisely is the aim of Yoga, — to get out of the cycle of Karma into a divine movement.

KARMA YOGA

I do not know why you drag in humanitarianism, activism, philanthropical seva etc. None of these are part of my Yoga or in harmony with my works, so they don't touch me. I never thought that politics or feeding the poor or writing beautiful poems would lead straight to Vaikuntha or the Absolute. It is not the form of the work itself or mere activity but the consciousness and Godward will behind it that are the essence of Karmayoga.

*

To do work in a close union and deep communion with the Divine in us, the Universal around us and the Transcendent above us, not to be shut up any longer in the imprisoned and separative human mind, the slave of its ignorant dictates and narrow suggestions, this is Karmayoga.

*

To work in obedience to a divine command, an eternal will, a universal impulse initiated by a transcendent compulsion, not to run under the whips of ego and need and passion and desire, and not to be guided by the pricks of mental and vital and physical preferences, but to be moved by God only, by the highest Truth only, this is Karmayoga.

LIFE (ORDINARY AND SPIRITUAL)

One who has not the courage to face patiently and firmly life and its difficulties will never be able to go through the still greater inner difficulties of the sadhana. The very first lesson in this Yoga is to face life and its trials with a quiet mind, a firm courage and an entire reliance on the Divine Shakti.

*

The life of *saṁsāra* is in its nature a field of unrest — to go through it in the right way one has to offer one's life and actions to the Divine and pray for the peace of the Divine within. When the mind becomes quiet, one can feel the Divine Mother supporting the life and put everything into her hands.

*

All the insistence upon action is absurd if one has not the light by which to act. "Yoga must include life and not exclude it" does not mean that we are bound to accept life as it is with all its stumbling ignorance and misery and the obscure confusion of human will and reason and impulse and instinct which it expresses.

One must go deep and find the soul, the self, the Divine Reality within us and only then can life become a true expression of what we can be.

*

Divinisation itself does not mean the destruction of the human elements; it means taking them up, showing them the way to their own perfection, raising them by purification and perfection to their full power and Ananda and that means the raising of the whole of earthly life to its full power and Ananda.

*

It is a lesson of life that always in this world everything fails a man — only the Divine does not fail him, if he turns entirely to the Divine.

*

Everything depends upon the aim you put before you. If, for the realisation of one's spiritual aim, it is necessary to give up the ordinary life of the Ignorance, it must be done; the claim of the ordinary life cannot stand against that of the spirit.

*

In the Yoga practised here the aim is to rise to a higher consciousness and to live out of the higher consciousness alone, not with the ordinary motives. This means a change of life as well as a change of consciousness. But all are not so circumstanced that they can cut loose from the ordinary life; they accept it therefore as a field of experience and self-training in the earlier stages of the sadhana. But they must take care to look at it as a field of experience only and to get free from the ordinary desires, attachments and ideas which usually go with it; otherwise, it becomes a drag and hindrance on their sadhana. When one is not compelled by circumstances there is no necessity to continue the ordinary life.

*

It is quite possible for you to do sadhana at home and in the midst of your work. What is necessary at the beginning is to remember the Mother as much as possible, to concentrate on her in the heart for a time every day, if possible, thinking of her as the Divine Mother, to aspire to feel her there with you, offer her your works and pray that from within she may guide and sustain you. This is a preliminary stage which often takes long, but if one goes through it with sincerity and steadfastness, the mentality begins little by little to change and a new consciousness opens in the sadhak which begins to be aware more and more of the Mother's presence within, of her working in the nature and in the life.

*

Peace is never easy to get in the life of the world and never constant, unless one lives deep within and bears the external activities as only a surface front of being.

*

Cases are seen in which the predictions of the horoscope fulfil themselves with great accuracy up to a certain age, then apply no more. This often happens when the subject turns away from the ordinary life to the spiritual life. If the turn is very radical, the cessation of predictability may be immediate.

*

The question about the family duties can be answered in this way — the family duties exist so long as one is in the ordinary consciousness of the *gṛhastha*; if the call to a spiritual life comes, whether one keeps to them or not depends partly upon the way of Yoga one follows, partly on one's own spiritual necessity.

*

When one has to escape from the lower dharma, one has often to renounce it so as to arrive at a larger one, i.e., social duties, paying debts, looking after family, help to serve your country, etc. etc. The man who turns to the spiritual life, has to leave all that behind him and often he is reproached by lots of people for his adharma. But if he does not do this adharma, he is bound for ever to the lower life — for there is always some duty there to be done — and cannot take up the spiritual dharma ever.

*

In the worldly life, the one thing by which one can enter into the sadhana is to remember the Divine always, taking one's difficulties as ordeals to be passed through, to pray constantly and seek the Divine help and protection and ask for the opening of the heart and consciousness to the supporting Divine Presence.

*

A divine life upon earth, the ideal we have placed before us, can only come about by a spiritual change of our being and a radical and fundamental change, an evolution or revolution of our nature. The embodied being upon earth would have to rise out of the domination over it of its veils of mind, life and body into the full consciousness and possession of its spiritual reality and its nature also would have to be lifted out of the consciousness and power of consciousness proper to mental, vital and physical being into the greater consciousness and greater power of being and the larger and freer life of the spirit.

The Mother:

The aim of ordinary life is to carry out one's duty, the aim of spiritual life is to realise the Divine.

*

It is the Spirit, the spiritual consciousness and the divine Presence that give life all its value; without this spiritual consciousness and this divine Presence life has no value....

This means that from the point of view of the truth of things, a man who has no material possessions, no remarkable capacity or possibility but is conscious of his psychic being and united with the Divine in him is infinitely greater than a ruler of the earth or a millionaire possessing considerable material power but unconscious of his psychic being.

From the point of view of truth, things apparent and external have no true value. The only thing that has a value is the divine Consciousness and the union with the Spirit....

The true spiritual life begins when one is in communion with the Divine, in the psychic....

When one is united with one's psychic being and conscious of the divine Presence, when one gets the impulse for action from this divine presence, when one's will has become a conscious collaborator with the divine will, then that is the starting-point.

Before this, one can be an aspirant for the spiritual life, but has not got the true spiritual life.

LOVE (HUMAN AND DIVINE)

As for love, the love must be turned singly towards the Divine. What men call by the name is a vital interchange for mutual satisfaction of desire, vital impulse or physical pleasure.

*

The whole principle of this Yoga is to give oneself entirely to the Divine alone and to nobody and nothing else, and to bring down into ourselves by union with the Divine Mother-Power all the transcendent light, force, wideness, peace, purity, truth-consciousness and Ananda of the supramental Divine. In this Yoga, therefore, there can be no place for vital relations or interchanges with others; any such relation or interchange immediately ties down the soul to the lower consciousness and its lower nature, prevents the true and full union with the Divine and hampers both the ascent to the supramental Truth-consciousness and the descent of the supramental Ishwari Shakti. Still worse would it be if this interchange took the form of a sexual relation or a sexual enjoyment, even if kept free from any outward act; therefore these things are absolutely forbidden in the sadhana.

*

Human love is mostly vital and physical with a mental support — it can take an unselfish, noble and pure form and expression only if it is touched by the psychic. One who wishes to reach the Divine must not burden himself with human loves and attachments, for they form so many fetters and hamper his steps, turning him away besides from the concentration of his emotions on the one supreme object of love. One must also be on one's guard against the profession of psychic love when one is doing sadhana, — for that is most often a cloak and justification for yielding to a vital attraction or attachment.

*

To run about expressing love for one's personal satisfaction or the satisfaction of others is only to spoil and lose it. One can love divinely only by becoming divine in nature; there is no other way.

The true love for the Divine is a self-giving, free of demands, full of submission and surrender, it makes no claim, imposes no condition, strikes no bargain, indulges in no violences of jealousy or pride or anger — for these things are not in its composition. Keep your love pure of all selfish claim and desire; you will find that you are getting all the love that you can bear and absorb in answer.

The Divine Love, unlike the human, is deep and vast and silent; one must become quiet and wide to be aware of it and reply to it. To give oneself is the secret of sadhana, not to demand and acquire. The more one gives oneself, the more the power to receive will grow. But for that all impatience and revolt must go; all suggestions of not getting, not being helped, not being loved, going away, of abandoning life or the spiritual endeavour must be rejected.

*

But whatever love or goodwill the human feeling is always either based on or strongly mixed with ego, — that is why it cannot be pure. It is said in the Upanishad, "One does not love the wife for the sake of the wife", or the child or friend etc. as the case may be "but for one's sake one loves the wife". There is usually a hope of return, of benefit or advantage of some kind, or of certain pleasures and gratifications, mental, vital or physical that the person loved can give. Remove these things and the love very soon sinks, diminishes or disappears or turns into anger, reproach, indifference or even hatred.

*

To bring the Divine Love and Beauty and Ananda into the world is, indeed, the whole crown and essence of our Yoga. But it has always seemed to me impossible unless there comes as its support and foundation and guard the Divine Truth — what I call the Supramental — and its Divine Power. Otherwise Love itself blinded by the confusions of this present consciousness may stumble in its human receptacles and, even otherwise, may find itself unrecognised, rejected or rapidly degenerating and lost in the frailty of man's inferior nature.

*

Universal love is the spiritual, founded on the sense of the One and the Divine everywhere and the change of the personal into a wide universal consciousness, free from attachment and ignorance.

*

The supramental love means an intense unity of soul with soul, mind with mind, life with life, and an entire flooding of the body consciousness with the physical experience of oneness, the presence of the Beloved in every part, in every cell of the body.

The Mother:

The Divine Love of which I speak is a Love that manifests here upon this physical earth, in matter, but it must be pure of its human distortions, if it is to incarnate. But the adverse forces have distorted it; they have turned it into a field of violence and selfishness and desire and every kind of ugliness and prevented it from taking part in the divine work.

*

Love is a supreme force which the Eternal Consciousness sent down from itself into an obscure and darkened world that it might bring back that world and its beings to the Divine. The creation moves upward through love towards the Divine. This human movement of love is secretly seeking for something else than what it has yet found; but it does not know where to find it, it does not even know what it is. Once the creation is conscious, awakened, opened to love for the Divine, the Divine love pours itself without limit back into the creation; there is the joining of the extremes, supreme Spirit and manifesting Matter, and their divine union becomes constant and complete.

*

The Divine's Love is the power of Transformation. It has this power because it is for the sake of Transformation that it has given itself to the world and manifested everywhere. Not only into man but into all the atoms of Matter has it infused itself in order to bring the world back to the original Truth. The moment you open to it, you receive also its power of Transformation. What is essential is the true contact; for you will find that the true contact with it is sufficient to fill at once the whole of your being.

*

To love truly the Divine we must rise above attachments. To become conscious of the Divine Love, all other love must be abandoned.

*

There is always a bitter taste behind the human love — it is only the Divine Love which never disappoints. It is to the sincerity of your aspiration that the Love answers spontaneously.

*

Only he who loves can recognise love. Those who are incapable of giving themselves in a sincere love, will never recognise love anywhere, and the more the love is divine, that is to say unselfish, the less they can recognise it.

*

Devotion is love and respect plus consecration. Without self-giving there is no love. But self-giving is very very rare in human love which is full of selfishness. Even a baby's love is quite selfish, because it asks for something in exchange, but the so-called human love is much worse; it only wants to possess its object. Devotion is much superior to human love, it is the first step towards self-giving.

*

If it is divine Love you are speaking of, you can have it only by giving up human love which is its disguise and caricature.

*

Of all austerities, the most difficult is the austerity of feeling and emotion, the Tapasya of love.

*

In the name of love the worst crimes have been perpetrated, the wildest follies committed. And yet, man has invented all kinds of moral and social rules hoping to control this force of love, to make it sober and docile. For it is not by rules that the movements of love can be governed. Only a greater, higher and truer power of love can master the uncontrollable impulses of love. Love can alone rule over love by illumining, transforming and enlarging it.

*

Consciousness is indeed the creator of the universe, but love its saviour. The love, the thing to which human beings give that name, has suffered all the degradations and thus it has been lowered to the level of the beast.

*

In the human beings love is immediately mixed with the egoistic lower movements that tarnish it and take away all the power of its purity. The exceptional souls, who seek the spiritual progress towards the creation of a new race, the race that will express the supramental truth upon earth, have to reject all love that is between human beings; for, however beautiful and pure it is, it creates a kind of short circuit and cuts the direct connection with the Divine.

One who has known Divine Love, finds all other love obscure, mixed with smallness and egoism and darkness. It looks like a bargain or a struggle for superiority and authority: and even in the best, it is full of misunderstanding and sensitiveness, frictions and misgivings. Moreover, it is a well-known fact that you grow into the likeness of him whom you love. If you want to be like the Divine, love Him alone. It is this wonderful state that we wish to realise upon earth; it is this which will transform the world and make it a habitation worthy of the Divine Presence. He will be able to manifest himself in the plenitude of his perfection only when human beings have made some indispensable progress in their consciousness and in their body.

No effort, therefore, is too arduous, no austerity too rigorous, if it can illumine, purify, perfect and transform the physical substance so that it may no longer conceal the Divine, when the Divine takes in it an outward form. For that marvel of love will then freely express itself in the world, the love divine which has the power of changing life into a paradise of sweet joy.

Your joys and your pleasures you will await from the Divine alone. In Him alone you will seek and find help and support. He will comfort you in all your pain, lead you on the path, lift you up if you stumble, and if there are moments of faintness and exhaustion, he will take you in his strong arms of love and wrap you in his soothing sweetness.

MADNESS IN SADHANA

Those who fall into insanity have lost the true touch and got into the wrong contact. It is due either to some impurity and unspiritual desire with which the seeker enters into the way or some insincerity, egoism and false attitude or to some weakness in the brain or nervous system which cannot bear the Power it has called down into it.

*

If the being is small, the nature weak and incapable, there is not this large-scale disaster; but a loss of balance, a mental unhinging and fall into unreason or a vital unhinging and consequent moral aberration or a deviation into some kind of morbid abnormality of the nature may be the untoward consequence.

The Mother :

When people begin Yoga out of ambition or vanity, it very frequently happens that they put themselves under the influence of certain hostile forces.

MATERIALISM — SPIRITUALISM

Materialism can hardly be spiritual in its basis because its basic method is just the opposite of the spiritual way of doing things. The spiritual works from within outward, the way of materialism is to work from out inwards.

Materialism seeks to "perfect" humanity by outward means and one of the main efforts is to construct a perfect social machine which will train and oblige men to be what they ought to be. But spirituality can only come by opening of the mind, vital and physical to the inmost soul, to the higher Self, to the Divine, and their subordination to the spiritual forces and instrumentation as channels of the inner Light, the higher Knowledge and Power.

*

It is quite true that the word "superstition" has been habitually used as a convenient club to beat down any belief that does not agree with the ideas of the materialistic reason, that is to say, the physical mind dealing with the apparent law of physical process and seeing no further. It has also been used to dismiss ideas and beliefs not in agreement with one's own idea of what is the rational norm of supraphysical truths as well. Even in the field of supraphysical experience only so much was admitted as could give a mentally rational explanation of itself according to a certain range of idea — all the rest, everything that seemed to demand an occult, mystic or below-the-surface origin to explain it was put aside as so much superstition.

*

Why I call the materialist's denial an *a priori* denial is because he refuses even to consider or examine what he denies but starts by denying it like Leonard Woolf with his "quack, quack" on the ground that it contradicts his own theories, so it can't be true.

*

If one is blind, it is quite natural to deny daylight: if one's highest natural vision is that of glimmering mists, it is equally natural to believe that all high vision is but a mist or a glimmer. But Light exists for all that — and Spiritual Truth is more than a mist and a glimmer.

*

The so-called sciences which deal with the mind and men are so much dependent on physical science that they cannot go beyond their narrow limits. If science is to turn her face towards the Divine, it must be a new science not yet developed which deals directly with the forces of the life-world and of Mind and so arrives at what is beyond Mind; but present-day science cannot do that.

*

The soul is not divided from God by these barriers of material dimensions. What is true of matter is not true of Spirit, nor do the standards of form apply to the formless. For Matter is conscious being confined in form, the spirit is conscious being using form but not confined in it; and it is the privilege of spirit that though indivisible in its pure being, it is freely self-divisible in its conscious experience and can concentrate itself in many states at a time.

*

Even the truth of physical things cannot be entirely known, nor can the right use of our material existence be discovered by physical Science and an outward knowledge alone or made possible by the mastery of physical and mechanical processes alone: to know, to use rightly we must go beyond the truth of physical phenomenon and process, we must know what is within and behind it.

MATERIAL OBJECTS

It is very true that physical things have a consciousness within them which feels and responds to care and is sensitive to careless touch and rough handling. To know or feel that and learn to be careful of them is a great progress of consciousness. It is always so that the Mother has felt and dealt with physical things.

*

The rough handling and careless breaking or waste and misuse of physical things is a denial of the Yogic Consciousness and a great hindrance to the bringing down of the Divine Truth to the material plane.

*

There is a consciousness in physical things, a life which is not the life and consciousness of man and animal which we know, but still secret and real. That is why we must have a respect for physical things and use them rightly, not misuse and waste, ill-treat or handle with a careless roughness. This feeling of all being conscious or alive comes when our own physical consciousness — and not the mind only — awakes out of its obscurity and becomes aware of the One in all things, the Divine everywhere.

The Mother :

Yes, I am in things also and that is why they must be treated with care.

*

Not to take care of material things which one uses is a sign of inconscience and ignorance.

You have no right to use any material object whatsoever if you do not take care of it.

You must take care of it not because you are attached to it, but because it manifests something of the Divine Consciousness.

MONEY

Money is the visible sign of a universal force, and this force in its manifestation on earth works on the vital and physical planes and is indispensable to the fullness of the outer life. In its origin and its true action it belongs to the Divine. But like other powers of the Divine it is delegated here and in the ignorance of the lower Nature can be usurped for the uses of the ego or held by Asuric influences and perverted to their purpose. To reconquer it for the Divine to whom it belongs and use it divinely for the divine life is the supramental way for the Sadhaka. All wealth belongs to the Divine and those who hold it are trustees, not possessors.

The Mother :

A day shall come when all the wealth of this world, freed at last from the enslavement to the anti-divine forces, offers itself spontaneously and fully to the service of the Divine's Work upon earth.

*

Money is not a thing that can be acquired honestly and quickly at the same time.

Those who try to earn quick, generally lose their honesty and straightforwardness — this is a great evil, for honour and honesty are much more valuable than money.

MORALITY, ETHICS

The spiritual life (adhyatma jivan), the religious life (dharmic jivan) and the ordinary human life of which morality is a part are three quite different things and one must know which one desires and not confuse the three together.

The ordinary life is that of the average human consciousness separated from its own true self and from the Divine and led by the common habits of the mind, life and body which are the laws of the Ignorance. The religious life is a movement of the same ignorant human consciousness, turning or trying to turn away from the earth towards the Divine but as yet without knowledge and led by the dogmatic tenets and rules of some sect or creed which claims to have found the way out of the bonds of the earth-consciousness into some beatific Beyond. The religious life may be the first approach to the spiritual, but very often it is only a turning about in a round of rites, ceremonies and practices of set ideas and forms without any issue. The spiritual life, on the contrary, proceeds directly by a change of consciousness, a change from the ordinary consciousness, ignorant and separated from its true self and from God, to a greater consciousness in which one finds one's true being and comes first into direct and living contact and then into union with the Divine. For the spiritual seeker this change of consciousness is the one thing he seeks and nothing else matters.

Morality is a part of the ordinary life; it is an attempt to govern the outward conduct by certain mental rules or to form the character by these rules in the image of a certain mental ideal. The spiritual life goes beyond the mind; it enters into the deeper consciousness of the Spirit and acts out of the truth of the Spirit.

*

Yoga is not a thing of ideas but of inner spiritual experience. Merely to be attracted to any set of religious or spiritual ideas does not bring with it any realisation. Yoga means a change of consciousness; a mere mental activity will not bring a change of consciousness, it can only bring a change of mind.

*

The popular account of reincarnation and Karma is based on the mere mental assumption that the workings of Nature ought to be moral and proceed according to an exact morality of equal justice — a scrupulous, even mathematical law of reward and punishment or, at any rate, of results according to a human idea of right correspondence. But Nature is non-moral — she uses forces and processes moral, immoral and amoral pell-mell for working out her business. Nature in her outward aspect seems to care for nothing except to get things done — or else to make conditions for an ingenious variety of the play of life. Nature in her deeper aspect as a conscious spiritual Power is concerned with the growth, by experience, the spiritual development of the souls she has in her charge.

*

It is the same with the problem of the taking of animal life. In fact the right decision might vary in each case and depend on a knowledge which the human mind has not — and it might very well be said that until it has it, it has not the right to take life. It was some dim perception of this truth that made religion and ethics develop the law of Ahimsa — and yet that too becomes a mental rule which it is found impossible to apply in practice. And perhaps the moral of it all is that we must act from the best according to our lights in each case, as things are, but that the solution of these problems can only come by pressing forward towards a greater light, a greater consciousness in which the problems themselves, as now stated by the human mind, will not arise because we shall have a vision which will see the world in a different way and a guidance which at present is not ours. The mental or moral rule is a stop-gap which men are obliged to use, very uncertainly and stumblingly, until they can see things whole in the light of the spirit.

*

The principle of life which I seek to establish is spiritual. Morality is a question of man's mind and vital, it belongs to a lower plane of consciousness. A spiritual life therefore cannot be founded on a moral basis, it must be founded on a spiritual basis. This does not mean that the spiritual man must be immoral — as if there were no other law of conduct than the moral. The law of action of the spiritual consciousness is higher, not lower than the moral — it is founded on union with the Divine and living in the Divine Consciousness and its action is founded on obedience to the Divine Will.

*

A moral man may be chock-full of ego, an ego increased by his own goodness and rectitude. Freedom from ego is spiritually valuable because then one can be centred, no longer in one's personal self, but in the Divine.

*

All that belongs to the intellectual-ethical virtue-and sin dodge which is only a mental construction of practical value for the outward life but not a truth of real inner values.

*

The greatest difficulty of the sattwic man is the snare of virtue and self-righteousness, the ties of philanthropy, mental idealisation, family affections, etc.

*

Suffering is simply a natural consequence of past errors, not a punishment, just as a burn is the natural consequence of playing with fire. It is part of the experience by which the soul through its instruments learns and grows until it is ready to turn to the Divine.

The Mother:

No one has a right to sit in judgement over moral and social laws, unless he has taken his seat above them; one cannot abandon them, unless one replaces them by something superior, which is not so easy. The majority of those who reject human laws and proclaim their liberty and their decision to "live their own life" do so only in obedience to the most ordinary vital movements which they disguise and try to justify, if not to their own eyes, at least, to the eyes of others. They give a kick to morality, simply because it is a hindrance to the satisfaction of their instincts. The moral consciousness acts in the same way in the social body as tapasya in the spiritual domain.

*

There is a great difference between spirituality and morality, two things that are constantly confused with each other. The spiritual life has for its object to grow into the divine consciousness. Morality proceeds by mental constructions with the idea of good or bad and sets up an ideal type into which all must force themselves. This moral ideal differs in its constituents and its ensemble in different times and different places. And it proclaims itself as a unique type and it admits of none other outside itself.

Morality lifts up one artificial standard contrary to the variety of life and the freedom of the spirit. Morality is not divine or of the Divine; it is of man and human. But the spiritual life demands that you should reject desire altogether. Its law is that you must cast aside all movements that draw you away from the Divine. All desires, whether good or bad, come within the description; for desire itself arises from an unillumined vital being and its ignorance.

*

You can break moral rules only when you observe the divine Law.

MOTHER'S WORKING

The Mother deals with each one in a different way, according to their need and their nature, not according to any fixed mental rule. It would be absurd for her to do the same thing with everybody as if all were machines which had to be touched and handled in the same way. It does not at all mean that she has more affection for one than for another, or those she touches in a particular way are better sadhaks or less so. The sadhaks think in that way because they are full of ignorance and ego. Instead of thinking whether the Mother favours one more or the other less, comparing and watching what she does, they ought to be concerned at Pranam with only their own spiritual reception of her influence. Pranam is for that and not for these other things which have nothing to do with sadhana.

*

Jealousy and envy are things common to human nature, but these are the very things that a sadhak ought to throw out of himself. Otherwise why is he a sadhak at all? He is supposed to be here for seeking the Divine — but in the seeking for the Divine jealousy, envy, anger, etc. have no place. They are movements of the ego and can only create obstacles to the union with the Divine.

*

It is much better to remember that one is seeking for the Divine and make that the whole governing idea and aim of the life. It is that which pleases the Mother more than anything else; these jealousies and envies and competitions for her favour can only displease and distress her.

*

Mother's seriousness [at Pranam] is due to some absorption in some work she is doing or very often to some strong attack of hostile forces in the atmosphere. It is a mistake to think that the Mother's not smiling means either displeasure or disapproval of something wrong in the sadhak.

*

If any one is in serious trouble in the Ashram, that falls on us and most on the Mother — so it is absurd to suppose that we can take pleasure in anyone suffering.

*

The danger of helping others is the danger of taking upon oneself their difficulties. If Mother can keep herself separated and help, this does not occur. But the tendency in helping is to take the person partially or completely in one's larger self. This is what the Mother has had to do with the sadhaks and the reason why she has sometimes to suffer.

*

All bad thoughts upon the Mother or throwing of impurities on her may affect her body as she has taken the sadhaks into her consciousness; nor can she send these things back to them as it might hurt them.

*

If the Mother were able to bring out the Divine personalities and Powers into her body and physical being as she was doing for several months without break some years ago, the brightest period in the history of the Ashram, things would be much more easy and all these dangerous attacks that now take place would be dealt with rapidly and would in fact be impossible. In those days when the Mother was either receiving the sadhaks for meditation or otherwise working and concentrating all night and day without sleep and very irregular food, there was no ill-health and no fatigue in her and things were proceeding with a lightning swiftness. The power used was not that of the Supermind, but of the Overmind, but it was sufficient for what was being done. Afterward because the lower vital and the physical of the sadhaks could not follow, the Mother had to push the Divine personalities and Powers through which she was doing the action behind a veil and came down into the physical human level and act according to its conditions and that means difficulties, struggles, illness, ignorance and inertia. But for the advance to be anything like general or swift in its process, the attitude of the sadhaks, not of a few only, must change. They must cling less to the conditions and feelings of the external physical consciousness and open themselves to the true consciousness of the Yogin and sadhak. If they did that, the inner eye would open and they would not be bewildered or alarmed if the Mother again manifested externally something of the Divine Personalities and Powers as she did before. They would not be asking her to be always on their level, but would be glad to be drawn swiftly or gradually up towards her. The difficulties would be ten times less and a larger, easier, securer movement possible.

*

Things are no longer what they were before when you were here. At that time the Mother was bringing down a rapid (collective as well as individual) transformation and creation into the mental, vital and physical planes from above, by the power of a supra-mental light and force acting through the higher illumined mind and the psychic being. For that purpose she was calling down beings of higher plane (like the one of which you speak) as an indispensable aid in that process. All went well enough so long as the work was on the mental, psychic and higher vital levels. But as soon as it began in the lower vital, it appeared at once that the lower vital and physical nature of human beings (at least of those here) were too small, obscure and full of rebellious impurity to admit of so great a working. One after another failed in the test and you were among the first to fall. The creation had to be postponed, the process changed and instead of doing all from above it became necessary to come down into the lower vital and inanimate nature for a long, slow, patient and difficult work of opening and change.

*

It is not by his own strength or good qualities that any one can attain the divine change; there are only two things that matter, the Mother's force at work and the sadhak's will to open to it and trust in her working. Be sure that the Mother will always be with you to carry you upon the path. Difficulties come and difficulties go, but she being with you, the victory is sure.

*

Always calls of this kind are coming to the Mother, sometimes a hundred close upon each other and always the answer is given. The occasions are of all kinds, but whatever the need that occasions the call, the Force is there to answer it. That is the principle of this action on the occult plane. It is not of the same kind as an ordinary human action and does not need a written or oral communication on the one who calls; an interchange of psychic communication is quite sufficient to set the Force at work. At the same time it is not an impersonal Force and the suggestion of a divine energy that is there ready to answer and satisfy anybody who calls it is not at all relevant here. It is something personal to the Mother and if she had not this power and this kind of action she would not be able to do her work.

*

The Mother has made an arrangement with a view to all the occult forces and the best possible conditions for the protection of the sadhaks from certain forces of death, diseases, etc. It cannot work perfectly because the sadhaks themselves have not the right attitude towards food and kindred vital physical things. But still there is a protection. If, however, the sadhaks go outside her formation, it must be on their own responsibility. But this arrangement is for the Ashram and not for those who are outside.

*

When the pressure of the Mother's Force works upon the consciousness, then in the plane on which it happens to be working, a great activity of different forces is set in play, e.g. if it is the mind, various mental forces, if it is the vital, various vital forces. It is not safe to take all these for true things, to be accepted without question and followed as commands of the Mother. No voice heard within can prevail against her word and no intimation that comes through your mind can be accepted as binding unless it is confirmed by her.

*

It is the emanation of the Mother that is with each sadhak all the time. In former days when she was spending the night in a trance and not working in the Ashram, she brought back with her the knowledge of all that was happening to everybody. Nowadays she has no time for that.

*

The Emanation is not a deputy, but the Mother herself. She is not bound to her body, but can put herself out (emanate) in any way she likes. What emanates, suits itself to the nature of the personal relation she has with the sadhak which is different with each, but that does not prevent it from being herself.

*

An emanation or a part of Her being and consciousness comes out of the Mother to each sadhak and as Her image and representative remains with him to help him. In fact, it is the Mother Herself who comes out in that form.

*

Mother's contact is there all the day and the night also. If one keeps the right contact with her inwardly all day, the Pranam will bear its right fruit, for you will be in the right condition to receive. I mean the inner contact in which one either feels one with her or in contact with her or aware of her presence or at the very least turned towards her always.

OCCULTISM

Occult forces are the forces that can only be known by going behind the veil of apparent phenomena — especially the forces of the subtle physical and supraphysical planes.

Such a seeking for occult powers is looked on with disfavour for the most part by spiritual teachers in India, because it belongs to the inferior planes and usually pushes the seeker on a path which may lead him very far from the Divine. Especially a contact with the forces and beings of the astral (or, as we term it, the vital) plane is attended with great dangers. The beings of this plane are often hostile to the true aim of spiritual life and establish contact with the seeker and offer him powers and occult experiences only in order that they may lead him away from the spiritual path or else that they may establish their own control over him or take possession of him for their own purpose. Often, representing themselves as divine powers, they mislead, give erring suggestions and impulsions and pervert the inner life. This is one of the chief dangers of the spiritual life and to be on one's guard against it is a necessity for the seeker if he wishes to arrive at his goal. It is true that many supraphysical or supernormal powers come with the expansion of the consciousness in Yoga but these powers are not sought after, they come naturally, and they have not the astral character. Also, they have to be used on purely spiritual lines, that is by the Divine Will and the Divine Force, as an instrument, but never as an instrumentation of the forces and beings of the vital plane.

*

Our object is not to get powers, but to ascend towards the divine Truth-Consciousness and bring its Truth down into the lower members. With the Truth all the necessary powers will come, not as one's own, but as the Divine's. The contact with the Truth cannot grow through rajasic mental and vital self-assertion, but only through psychic purity and surrender.

The Mother :

To talk about occult things is of little value; one must experience them. It is a system of knowledge organised around some principles; it follows a precise process and if you reproduce exactly the same conditions, you get always the same results. It is also a progressive knowledge. Only this study deals with realities which do not belong to the most material world.

As we possess a physical body, so we possess also other more subtle bodies with their own senses, but more refined, more precise, much more powerful than our physical senses. Naturally, as our education is not accustomed to deal with this domain, these senses are usually not developed and the worlds where they function escape our ordinary consciousness; yet children spontaneously live a great deal in this domain. It is only with an intensive mental development that these capacities fade away in children and often end by disappearing altogether.

In all ages, there were upon earth isolated individuals or small groups; they used to practise this type of science. They sought for especially gifted souls and gave them the necessary training. Usually these groups lived a more or less secret or hidden life because ordinary people are very intolerant of this kind of capacities and activities which pass their understanding and frighten them.

In all the domains of human activity, there are charlatans and imposters. But the fraud practised by them should not throw discredit upon a true science which they falsely boast they possess. That is why in the great epochs when this science flourished, when there were recognised schools where it was practised, whoever wanted to undertake this study, before being admitted, was made to go through, for a long time, sometimes even for years, a two-fold discipline of a very strict nature, that of self-development and self-mastery. In this way the height and nobility of the candidate's aspiration was proved.

Occult science, in one of its aspects, is something of chemistry applied to the play of forces, the building of worlds and individual forms in inner dimensions. As in the chemistry of Matter, the handling of certain substances is not without danger, even so in the occult worlds the handling of certain forces and contact with them involve risks which can prove harmless only if one keeps a cool head and unshakable calm.

In any case, at all times it has been recommended that one should take up these studies only under a sure guide who can point out the path to follow, put you on guard against dangers, whether illusory or not and give protection when needed.

Occult knowledge without the spiritual discipline is, if it falls into impure hands, a dangerous instrument for one who uses it as well as for others. Spiritual knowledge without the occult science lacks in precision and certainty in its objective effects : it is all-powerful only in the subjective world. The two, when combined whether for external or for internal action, are irresistible and become an instrument fit for the manifestation of the Supramental Power.

OCCULT HISTORY OF MAN

The Mother:

At the beginning of creation, four individual formations — the first personalities — made their appearance. They were : (1) a Being of Light or Consciousness, (2) a Being of Truth or Reality, (3) a Being of Love or Ananda and (4) a Being of Life. And the first law of creation was freedom of decision. These Beings were manifestations in the free movement of the Divine; they themselves moved free, according to their individualised conscious will. Soon, however, they stood out no longer on the Divine, but moved out of him, away and separate; they sought to fulfil their individualised will and destiny. The first fruit, the inevitable reaction of freedom was precisely a separation from the Divine, each one encircled within its ego, limited and bound to its own fund of potency: individualism means limitation and the Four Independants lapsed into their opposites: Light changed to Darkness, i.e. Consciousness to Unconsciousness, Truth changed to Falsehood, Delight changed to Pain and Suffering, and Life changed to Death. That is how the four undivine principles, the Powers of the Undivine came to rule and fashion the material creation.

Into the heart of this Darkness and Falsehood and Pain and Death, a seed was sown, a grain that is to be the epitome and symbol of material creation and in and through which the Divine will claim back all the elements gone astray, the prodigal ones who will return to recognise and fulfil the Divine. That was Earth. And the earth, in her turn, in her labour towards the Divine Fulfilment, out of her bosom, threw up a being who would again symbolise and epitomise the earth and material creation. That is Man. For, man came with the soul in him, the Psychic Being, the Divine Flame, the spark of consciousness in the midst of universal unconsciousness, a miniature of the original Divine Light-Truth-Love-Life.

*

I must tell you that the origin of these beings is prior to that of the gods; they are the first emanations, the first individual beings of the universe; so they cannot be got rid of so easily, by winning one battle [with Hitler].

They will exist so long as they are necessary for the universal evolution. The day they lose their utility, they will be converted or will disappear.

Besides, they know that they are nearing their last hour and that is why they are doing as much havoc as they can.

They are four. The first one has been converted, another is dissolved into its origin. Two are still living and these two are more stubborn than all the others. One is known in occultism as the "Lord of Falsehood", I have told you, the other is the Lord of Death. And as long as these two beings exist, there will be difficulties.

PHILOSOPHY

The Divine is not bound by human philosophies — it is free in its play and free in its essence.

*

Logic is the worst enemy of Truth, as self-righteousness is the worst enemy of virtue; for the one cannot see its own errors nor the other its own imperfections.

Philosophy is only a play of phrases and mental ideas — a mental gymnastic without any reference to experience. Spiritual knowledge is as much impossible without experience as scientific knowledge.

Philosophy is of little help in getting true knowledge, which must come from experience and actual realisation. It serves as a mental exercise — it makes the mind supple and clear; it gives ideas to the mind that there is something higher than itself to which it should aspire; thus it serves as a sort of springing-board.

The Mother:

The mistake is to look at things through the dimensions of the human consciousness. It is dangerous to try to explain or understand them with the limited mental intelligence. That is the reason why philosophy has always failed to unveil the secret of things; it is because it has tried to fit the universe into the size of the human mind.

THE PROBLEM OF WOMAN

The Mother:

No law can liberate women unless they liberate themselves. What makes them slaves is:—

(1) Attraction towards the male and his strength,
(2) Desire for home life and its security,
(3) Attachment to motherhood.

If they get free from these three slaveries, they will truly be the equal of men.

Men also have three slaveries:—

(1) Spirit of possession, attachment to power and domination,
(2) Desire for sexual relation with woman,
(3) Attachments to the small comforts of married life.

If they get rid of these three slaveries, they can truly become the equal of women.

*

Man feels himself superior and wants to dominate, the woman feels oppressed and revolts, openly or secretly; and the eternal quarrel between the sexes continues from age to age, identical in essence, innumerable in its forms and shades.

It is well understood that man throws the whole blame upon the woman, as woman in the same way throws the entire blame upon man. In truth the blame should be equally distributed between the two and neither should boast as being superior to the other. Moreover, as long as this notion of superiority and inferiority is not eliminated, nothing or nobody can put an end to the misunderstanding that divides the human race into two opposite camps and the problem will not be solved. In their mutual relations, man and woman are, at once and towards each other, quite despotic masters and somewhat pitiable slaves.

Yes, slaves; for so long as you have desires and preferences and attachments, you are a slave of these things and of those persons on whom you depend for their fulfilment.

That is why no law can liberate women unless they free themselves: men too, likewise, cannot, in spite of all their habits of domination, cease to be slaves unless they are freed from all their inner slavery.

This state of secret conflict, often not admitted, but always present in the subconscious, even in the best cases, seems inevitable, unless human beings rise above their ordinary consciousness to identify themselves with the perfect consciousness, to be unified with the supreme Reality. For when you attain this higher consciousness you perceive that the difference between man and woman reduces itself to a difference purely physical.

We dream of a world in which all these oppositions will at last disappear, where a being will be able to live and prosper who will be the harmonious synthesis of all that is best in human production, identifying conception and execution, vision and creation in one single consciousness and action.

In any case until the appearance of a new conception and a new consciousness compelling Nature to create a new race which will have no need any more to submit to the necessity of animal procreation and will not be under the compulsion of being cut into two complementary sexes, the best that can be done for the progress of the present human race is to treat the two sexes on a footing of perfect equality, to give both one and the same education and training and to teach them to find, through a constant contact with a Divine Reality which is above all sexual differentiation, the source of all possibilities and all harmonies.

And perhaps India, the land of contrasts, will also be the land of new realisations, even as she was the cradle of their conception.

READING

To read what will help the Yoga or what will be useful for the work or what will develop the capacities for the divine purpose. Not to read worthless stuff or for mere entertainment or for a dilettante intellectual curiosity which is out of the nature of a mental dram-drinking. When one is established in the highest consciousness, one can read nothing or everything; it makes no difference.

*

It is not by reading books that the mind is cultured — it is by trying to think and see things clearly that it comes. Reading is a quite secondary thing. One may read thousands of books, yet remain narrow and foolish.

*

You may have all the mental knowledge in the world and yet be impotent to face vital difficulties. Courage, faith, sincerity towards the Light, rejection of opposite suggestions and adverse voices are there the true help. Then only can knowledge itself be at all effective.

*

It is not reading that brings the contact with the Divine, it is the will and aspiration in the being that brings it.

*

What is written for X is not meant for you. He has got into a movement of consciousness in which reading is no longer necessary and would rather interfere with his consciousness. There is no objection to your reading provided it does not interfere with your meditation....

There should be no "desire" to be a "great" writer. If there is a genuine inspiration or coming of power to write then it can be done, but to use it as a means of service for the Divine is the proper spirit....

It depends upon what kind of 'literary man' you want to be, ordinary or yogic.

A literary man is one who loves literature and literary activity for its own sake. A yogic 'literary' man is not a literary man at all, but one who writes only what the inner will and Word wants to express. He is a channel and an instrument of something greater than his own literary personality....

It is the same with the work — it has a value of moral training, discipline, obedience, acceptance of work for the Mother. The spiritual value and result come afterwards when the consciousness in the vital opens upward. So with the mental work. It is a preparation....

RELIGION

Religion is always imperfect because it is a mixture of man's spirituality with his endeavours that come in in trying to sublimate ignorantly his lower nature.

*

Religions at the best modify only the surface of the nature. Moreover, they degenerate very soon into a routine of ceremonial habitual worship and fixed dogmas.

*

Religion in fact is not knowledge, but a faith and aspiration; it is justified indeed both by an imprecise intuitive knowledge of large spiritual truths and by the subjective experience of souls that have risen beyond the ordinary life, but in itself it only gives us the hope and faith by which we may be induced to aspire to the intimate possession of the hidden tracts and larger realities of the Spirit. That we turn always the few distinct truths and the symbols or the particular discipline of a religion into hard and fast dogmas, is a sign that as yet we are only infants in the spiritual knowledge and are yet far from the science of the Infinite.

*

Going for pilgrimage to holy places has nothing to do with the Truth; it is a religious exercise for the people of ordinary consciousness.

The Mother:

Religion belongs to the higher mind of humanity. It is the effort of man's higher mind to approach, as far as lies in its power, something beyond it, to which humanity gives the name of God, which the human mind cannot reach and yet tries to reach. Religion may be divine in its ultimate origin but in its actual nature it is not divine but human. The religions made by man are many and most of them have been made in the same way. We know how the Christian religion came into existence. It was certainly not Jesus who made what is known as Christianity, but some learned and very clever men put their heads together and built it up into the thing we see. There was nothing divine in the way in which it was formed, and there is nothing divine either in the way in which it functions.

Buddha discovered a way out of earthly suffering and misery. He saw a Truth which he endeavoured to express and communicate to the disciples and followers who gathered around him. But even before he was dead, his teaching had already begun to be twisted and distorted. After his disappearance Buddhism as a full-fledged religion reared its head, founded upon what the Buddha is supposed to have said and on the supposed significance of these reported sayings. Later on the disciples could not agree on what the Master had said and there grew up a host of sects and sub-sects in the body of the parent-religion, each of them claiming to be the only, the original, the undefiled doctrine of the Buddha. The same fate overtook the teaching of the Christ. All religions have each the same story to tell. The Teacher comes and reveals the Truth but men seize upon it, trade upon it, make an almost political organisation out of it.

The first and principal article of these established and formal religions runs always, "Mine is the supreme, the only truth, all others are in falsehood or inferior". For without this fundamental dogma, established credal religions could not have existed. If you do not believe and proclaim that you alone possess the one or the highest truth, you will not be able to impress people and make them flock to you.

The articles and dogmas of a religion are mind-made things and if you cling to them and shut yourself up in a code of life made out for you, you would not know and cannot know the truth of the Spirit that lies beyond all codes and dogmas, wide and large and free. When you stop at a religious creed and tie yourself in it, taking it for the only truth in the world, you stop the advance and widening of your inner soul. For some natures religion has a use and it is even necessary to them; for, through external forms, like the ceremonies of the Church, it offers a kind of support and help to their inner spiritual aspiration. For them religion is not an obstacle; an obstacle for those who can go farther. All countries and all religions are built up out of a mass of traditions. You will then perceive what a mockery it is to say, "Because I am brought up in this religion, therefore it is the only true religion: because I am born in this country, therefore it is the best of all countries".

Things have an inner value and become real to you, only when you have acquired them by the exercise of your free choice, not when they have been imposed upon you. Then only you can say with an inner truth, "This is my family, this my country, this my religion".

Each of us has been born in many different countries, belonged to many different nations, followed many different religions. Why must we accept the last one as the best?

If your aim is to be free, in the freedom of the Spirit, you must get rid of all the ties that are not the inner truth of your being. There can be no such imposition in your relation with the Divine. Truth is self-evident and has not to be imposed upon the world. It does not feel the need of being accepted by men; for it is self-existent. But one who is founding a religion needs to have many followers. The greatness of spiritual truth is not in numbers. The average man is drawn towards those who make great pretensions and those who make great pretensions need to proclaim loudly and to advertise; for otherwise they would not attract great numbers of people.

*

When you come to the Yoga, you must be ready to have all your mental buildings and all your vital scaffoldings shattered to pieces. You must be prepared to be suspended in the air with nothing to support you except your faith. You will have to forget your past self and its clingings altogether, to pluck it out of your consciousness and be born anew, free from every kind of bondage. Think not of what you were, but of what you aspire to be; be all in what you want to realise. Turn from your dead past and look straight towards the future. Your religion, country, family lie there; it is the DIVINE ALONE.

Visiting of Holy Places, Temples, Churches etc.

The Mother:

People of ordinary consciousness take to the thing through a kind of superstition; one thinks, "if I go to the temple or to the Church once a week, for example, if I say my prayers regularly, something good will happen to me." It is a superstition spread all over the world, but it has no spiritual value....

I have been to holy places. I have seen monuments considered as very highly religious, in France, Japan and elsewhere; they were not always the same kind of temples or churches nor were they the same gods but the impression they left on me, my experiences of them were everywhere almost the same, with but slight differences. For instance, in a most famous and most beautiful place of worship, I saw within its holy of holies a huge black Spider that had spread its net all around, caught within it and absorbed all the energies emanating from the devotion of the people, their prayers and all that. It was not a very pleasant spectacle. Now if I had gone and told them: you think it is God you are praying to! it is only a formidable vital Spider that is sucking your force. Surely it would not have been very charitable on my part. But everywhere it is almost the same thing. There is a vital Force presiding. And vital beings feed upon the vibrations of human emotion. Very few are they, a microscopic number, who go to the temples and churches and holy places with the true religious feeling, not to pray or beg something of God, but to offer themselves, to express gratitude, to aspire, to surrender. These when they are there, get some touch of the Divine just for the moment. But all others go only out of superstition, egoism, self-interest and create the atmosphere as it is found and it is that you usually breathe in when you go to a holy place....

I have purposely made the experiment a little everywhere. Almost everywhere it is but a web of adverse vital forces that use everything for their food. The bigger the congregation, the more portentous the vital deity. Besides, in the invisible world it is only the vital beings that like to be worshipped. When they can have a troop of people adoring them, they reach the very height of satisfaction....

But if you take a truly divine being, that is not the thing he likes or appreciates. He does not like to be worshipped; worship does not give him special pleasure. But if he sees anywhere a fine intuitive sense, a good feeling, a movement of unselfishness or spiritual enthusiasm, he considers that as infinitely more valuable than prayers and Pujas. He feels neither flattered nor satisfied nor glorified by your Puja....

From this standpoint it is good that for a time humanity should come out of the religious atmosphere, full of fear and blind superstitious submission by which the adverse forces have profited so monstrously. The age of negation, of atheism and positivism is from this view quite indispensable for man's liberation from sheer ignorance. It is only when you have come out of this, this abject submission to the evil forces of the Vital that you can rise to truly spiritual heights and then become their collaborators and right instruments for the forces of the Truth and Consciousness and Power. The superstitions of the lower levels you must leave far behind to rise high.

SPIRITUAL FORCE

All I can do is to send you the Force that if received would help you to change your condition; it is what I have always done. But it cannot act effectively — or at least not at once — if the doors are shut against it.

*

The outward touch is helpful; but the inward is still more helpful when one is accustomed to receive it with a certain concreteness — and the outward touch is not always fully possible, while the inward can be there all the time.

*

Certainly, my force is not limited to the Ashram and its conditions. As you know it is being largely used for helping the right development of the war and of change in the human world. It is also used for individual purposes outside the scope of the Ashram and the practice of Yoga; but that, of course, is silently done and mainly by a spiritual action. The Ashram, however, remains at the centre of the work and without the practice of Yoga the work would not exist and could not have any meaning or fruition.

*

It is not very advisable to discuss either myself or the Ashram or spiritual things with hostile minds or unbelievers. These discussions usually bring on the sadhak a stress of the opposing atmosphere and cannot be helpful to his progress. Reserve is the best attitude; one need not be concerned to dispel their bad will or their ignorance.

*

The Mother or myself send a force. If there is no openness, the force may be thrown back or return (unless we put a great force which is not advisable to do) as from an obstruction or resistance; if there is some openness, the result may be partial or slow; if there is the full openness or receptivity, then the result may be immediate. Of course, there are things that cannot be removed all at once, being an old part of the nature, but with receptivity these also can be more effectively and rapidly dealt with. Some people are so open that even by writing they get free before the book or letter reaches us.

*

The Yoga-force is always tangible and concrete in the way I have described and has tangible results. But it is invisible — not like a blow given or the rush of a motor car knocking somebody down which the physical senses can at once perceive. How is the mere physical mind to know that it is there and working? By its results? but how can it know that the results were that of the Yogic force and not of something else? One of the two things it must be. Either it must allow the consciousness to go inside, to become aware of inner things, to believe in the experience of the invisible and the supraphysical, and then by experience, by the opening of new capacities, it becomes conscious of these forces and can see, follow and use their workings just as the Scientist uses the unseen forces of Nature.

*

If you have spiritual force, it can act on people thousands of miles away who do not know and never will know that you are acting on them or that they are being acted upon — they only know that there is a force enabling them to do things and may very well suppose it is their own great energy and genius.

Spiritual force has its own concreteness; it can take a form of which one is aware and can send it quite concretely on whatever object one chooses.

*

I believe that all Yogins who have these powers do use them whenever they find that they are called on from within to do so. They may refrain if they think the use in a particular case is contrary to the Divine Will, or see that preventing one evil may be opening the door to worse or for any other valid reason, but not from any general prohibitory rule. What is forbidden to anyone with a strong spiritual sense is to be a miracle-monger, performing extraordinary things for show, for gain, for fame, out of vanity or pride. It is forbidden to use powers from mere vital motives, to make an Asuric ostentation of them or to turn them into a support for arrogance, conceit, ambition or any other of the amiable weaknesses to which human nature is prone. It is because half-baked Yogins so often fall into these traps of the hostile forces that the use of Yogic powers is something discouraged as harmful to the user.

*

I affirm again to you most strongly that this is the Mother's war [World War No. II]. You should not think of it as a fight for certain nations against others or even for India; it is a struggle for an ideal that has to establish itself on earth in the life of humanity, for a Truth that has yet to realise itself fully and against a darkness and falsehood that are trying to overwhelm the earth and mankind in the immediate future. It is the forces behind the battle that have to be seen and not this or that superficial circumstance.

*

Even if I knew that the Allies would misuse their victory or bungle the peace or partially at least spoil the opportunities open to the human world by that victory, I would still put my force behind them. At any rate things could not be one-hundreth part as bad as they would be under Hitler. The ways of the Lord would still be open and to keep them open is what matters.

*

Yoga develops power, it develops it even when we do not desire or consciously aim at it; and power is always a double-edged weapon which can be used to hurt or destroy as well as to help and save. Be it also noted that all destruction is not evil.

SUICIDE

Sadhana has to be done in the body, it cannot be done by the soul without the body. When the body drops, the soul goes wandering in other worlds — and finally it comes back to another life and another body. All the difficulties it had not solved meet it again in the new life. So what is the use of leaving the body?

Moreover, if one throws away the body wilfully, one suffers much in the other worlds and when one is born again, it is in worse, not in better conditions. The only sensible thing is to face the difficulties in this life and this body and conquer them.

*

Suicide is an absurd solution; he is quite mistaken in thinking that it will give him peace. He will only carry his difficulties with him into a more miserable condition of existence beyond and bring them back to another life on earth.

The Mother:

There are men who say, "How unhappy I am in this body", and think of death as an escape. But after death you have the same vital surroundings and are in danger from the same forces that are the cause of your misery in this life. The dissolution of the body forces you out into the open spaces of the vital world. And you have no longer a defence; there is not the physical body any longer to rush back to for safety.

It is here upon earth, in the body itself, that you must aquire a complete knowledge and learn to use a full and complete power. Only when you have done that will you be free to move about with entire security in all the worlds.

*

Know for certain that to commit suicide is the most foolish action that a man can do; because the end of the body does not mean the end of the consciousness and what was troubling you while you were alive continues to trouble you when you are dead, without the possibility of diverting your mind which you can get when you are alive.

*

It is *in this world* that you have to change and that the change is possible. If you run away from the world, you will have to come again probably in worse condition and you will have to do everything all over again.

It is much better not to be coward to think of suicide, but to face now the situation and to do the necessary effort to conquer.

SUPERMIND

Supermind is between the Sachchidananda and the lower creation. Supermind alone contains the self-determining Truth of the Divine Consciousness and is necessary for a Truth creation. One can of course realise Sachchidananda in relation to the mind, life and body also — but then it is something stable, supporting by its presence the lower Prakriti, but not transforming it. The Supermind alone can transform the lower nature.

All truths below the Supermind are either partial or relative or otherwise deficient and unable to transform the earthly life; they can only at most modify and influence it. The Supermind is the vast Truth-consciousness of which the ancient seekers spoke; there have been glimpses of it till now, sometimes an indirect influence of pressure, but it has not been brought down into the consciousness of the earth and fixed there. To so bring it down is the aim of our Yoga.

*

The Vedic Rishis never attained to the Supermind for the earth or perhaps did not even make the attempt. They tried to rise individually to the Supramental plane, but they did not bring it down and make it a permanent part of the earth-consciousness.

*

Our Yoga is a double movement of ascent and descent; one rises to higher and higher levels of consciousness, but at the same time one brings down their power not only into mind and life, but in the end even into the body. And the highest of these levels, the one at which it aims is the Supermind. Only when that can be brought down is a divine transformation possible in the earth-consciousness.

*

The Indian systems did not distinguish between two quite different powers and levels of consciousness, one which we can call Overmind and the other the true Supermind or Divine Gnosis. That is the reason why they got confused about Maya, and took it for the supreme creative power. In so stopping short at what was still a half-light they lost the secret of transformation, and concluded that the one thing to do was to get beyond it into some immovable and inactive silence of the Supreme.

*

Overmind stands at the top of the lower hemisphere, and you

have to pass through and beyond Overmind, if you would reach Supermind, while still above and beyond Supermind are the worlds of Sachchidananda.

*

But the last conversion is the supramental, for onc ethere — once the nature is supramentalised, we are beyond the Ignorance and conversion of consciousness is no longer needed, though a farther divine progression, even an infinite development is still possible.

*

In the Supramental consciousness there are no problems — the problem is created by the division set up by the Mind. The Supramental sees the Truth as a single whole and everything falls into its place in that whole.

*

Our aim is to bring the secret forces out and unwalled into the open, so that instead of getting some shadows or lightnings of themselves out through the veil or being wholly obstructed, they may pour down and flow in rivers.

One cannot get into the true Supermind unless one has first objectivised the overmind truth in life, speech, action, external knowledge and not only experienced it in meditation and inner experience.

*

It is quite impossible for the Supramental to take up the body before there has been the full supramental change in the mind and vital. Some people always expect some kind of miracle — they do not understand that it is a concentrated evolution, swift but following the law of creation that has to take place. A miracle can be a moment's wonder. A change according to the Divine Law can alone endure. The effect of the Supramental descent will create greater possibilities of advancing quickly in the sadhana than now.

*

The human physical is always full of dark, low and obscure forces. When the Supramental comes down fully into the material consciousness, it will create the right conditions there. The oneness will be created, the constant presence and sense of contact will be felt in the material and there will be all the actual physical contact that is needed.

Physical tamas in its roots can be removed only by the descent and the transformation, but physical exercise and regular activity of the body can always prevent a tamasic condition from prevailing in the body.

*

It is the supramental Power that transforms mind, life and body — not the Sachchidananda consciousness which supports impartially everything. But it is by having experience of the Sachchidananda, pure existence-consciousness-bliss, that the ascent to the supramental and the descent of the supramental become possible.

*

Nothing permanent can be done without the real Supramental Force. But the result of its descent would be that in human life intuition would become a greater and more developed force than it now is and the other intermediate powers between mind and Supermind would become also more common and develop an organised action.

*

Supermind is the grade of existence beyond mind, life and

Matter and, as mind, life and Matter have manifested on the earth, so too must Supermind in the inevitable course of things manifest in this world of Matter.

Its possession would enable the human being to rise beyond the normalities of his present thinking, feeling and being into those highest powers of the mind in its self-exceedings. Thus there will be built up, first, even in the Ignorance itself, the possibility of a human ascent towards a divine living.

*

Once the Supermind has descended upon a God-seeker and has the direction of his existence, all relations with the Divine will be his: the trinity of God-knowledge, divine works and devotion to God will open within him and move towards an utter self-giving and surrender of his whole being and nature. He will live in God and with God, possess God, even plunge in him forgetting all separate personality, but not losing it in self-extinction.

*

This world is, no doubt, based ostensibly upon Matter, but its summit is Spirit and the ascent towards Spirit must be the aim and justification of its existence and the pointer to its meaning and purpose. Therefore, if supermind exists, if it descends, if it becomes the ruling principle, all that seems impossible to mind becomes not only possible but inevitable.

*

No sadhak can reach the supermind by his own efforts and the effort to do it by personal tapasya has been the source of many mishaps. One has to go quietly stage by stage until the being is ready and even then it is only the Grace that can bring the real supramental change.

*

The Divine Force can act on any plane — it is not limited to the supramental Force. The Supramental is only one aspect of the power of the Divine.

*

Q : It is nearly 30 years since you started the work of bringing down the Supramental!

A : 30 years too little or too many? What would have satisfied your rational mind — 3 years? 3 months? 3 weeks? Considering that by ordinary evolution it could not have been done even at Nature's express speed in less than 3000 years, and would ordinarily have taken anything from 30,000 to 3,000,000, the transit of 30 years is perhaps not too slow.

*

It then becomes evident that the Overmind Power (in spite of its lights and splendours) is not sufficient to overcome the Ignorance because it is itself under the law of Division out of which came the Ignorance. One has to pass beyond and supramentalise Overmind so that mind and all the rest may undergo the final change.

*

It is only here that the Supramental Light can act for the present — in the places outside there is no preparation to receive it.... It is not possible for a force like the Supramental to come down without making a large change in earth conditions....It is first through the individuals that it becomes part of the earth-consciousness and afterwards it spreads from the first centres and takes up more and more of the global consciousness till it becomes an established force here.

*

As far as I can see, once the supramental is established in Matter, the transformation will be possible under much less troublesome conditions than now are there.

*

The supramental world has to be formed or created in us by the Divine Will as a result of a constant expansion and self-perfecting.

*

The supermind in its action is a thing of unity and harmony and inherent order. At first when the pressure from above falls on the mentality, this is not realised and even a contrary phenomenon may for a time appear. That is due to several causes. First, there may be a disturbance, even a derangement created by impact of the greater hardly measurable power on an inferior consciousness which is not capable of responding to it organically or even perhaps of bearing the pressure ... if the mind is not sufficiently passive and obedient to the higher guidance, may lead to a great excitation of power but also an increased disorder. It is for this reason that a previous preparation and long purification, the more complete the better, and a tranquillising and ordinarily a passivity of the mind calmly and strongly open to the spirit are necessities of the Yoga....

The Mother:

I do not see that the Supramental will act in the way you expect from it. Its action will be to effectuate the Divine's will upon the earth, whatever that may be. On men its action will be to turn their will consciously or unconsciously on their part towards the way in which the Divine's will wants to go.

THOUGHTS AND GLIMPSES

Because thou hast mistaken the instrument for the worker and the master and because thou seekest to choose by the ignorance of thy desire thy own state and thy own profit and thy own utility, therefore thou hast suffering and anguish and hast many times to be thrust into the red hell of the furnace and hast many times to be reborn and reshaped and retempered until thou shalt have learned thy human lesson. And all these things are because they are in thy unfinished nature.

*

The upward movement is the means towards fulfilment of existence in the world; the downward movement is destruction, Hell, perdition.

*

Life is supernatural to Matter, Mind supernatural to Life, ideal being supernatural to mental being, infinite being supernatural to ideal being. So too man is supernatural to the animal, God is supernatural to man. Man too as soon as he has assured his natural existence, must insist on his upward movement towards God. The upward movement towards Heaven, the downward movement towards Hell.

*

By yielding to Nature, we fall away both from Nature and from God; by transcending Nature we at once fulfil all the possibilities of Nature and rise towards God. The human touches first the divine and then becomes divine.

*

Not to be immersed, enmeshed and bound by Nature, not to

hate and destroy her, is the first thing we must learn if we would be complete Yogins and proceed towards our divine perfection. Perfect and comprehensive Yoga avoids limitation by aspects and leads to entire divinity.

*

If thou keepest this limited human ego and thinkest thyself the superman, thou art but the fool of thy own pride, the plaything of thy own force and the instrument of thy own illusions.

*

If thou canst not be the slave of all mankind, thou art not fit to be its master.

*

Only to those who have a true humility will power be given.

TRANSFORMATION

If you desire this transformation, put yourself in the hands of the Mother and her Powers without cavil or resistance and let her do unhindered her work within you. Three things you must have, consciousness, plasticity, unreserved surrender. But be on your guard and do not try to understand and judge the Divine Mother by your little earthly mind that loves to subject even the things that are beyond it to its own norms and standards, its narrow reasonings and erring impressions, its bottomless aggressive ignorance and its petty self-confident knowledge. The human mind shut in the prison of its half-lit obscurity cannot follow the many-sided freedom of the steps of the Divine Shakti. Open rather your soul to her and be content to feel her with the psychic nature and see her with the psychic vision that alone make a straight response to the Truth. Then the Mother herself will enlighten by their psychic elements your mind and heart and life and physical consciousness and reveal to them too her ways and her nature.

*

Transformation effected by the sadhana cannot be complete unless it is a supramentalisation of the being. Psychicisation is not enough, it is only a beginning; spiritualisation and the descent of the higher consciousness is not enough, it is only a middle term; the ultimate achievement needs the action of the Supramental Consciousness and Force. Something less than that may very well be considered enough by the individual, but it is not enough for the earth-consciousness to take the definitive stride forward.

*

If the transformation of the body is complete, that means no subjection to death — it does not mean that one will be bound to keep the same body for all time. One creates a new body for oneself when one wants to change, but how it will be done cannot be said now. The present method is by physical birth — some occultists suppose that a time will come when that will not be necessary — but the question must be left for the Supramental evolution to decide.

*

In the ordinary nature we live in the Ignorance and do not know the Divine. The forces of the ordinary nature are undivine Forces because they weave a veil of ego and desire and unconsciousness which conceals the Divine from us. To get into the higher and deeper consciousness which knows and lives consciously in the Divine, we have to get rid of the forces of the lower nature and open to the action of the Divine Shakti which will transform our consciousness into that of the Divine Nature.

*

Unless the external nature is transformed, one may go as high as possible and have the largest experiences, but the external mind remains an instrument of Ignorance.

*

There are different statuses of the divine consciousness. There are also different statuses of transformation. First is the psychic transformation, in which all is in contact with the Divine through the individual psychic consciousness. Next is the spiritual transformation in which all is merged in the Divine in the cosmic consciousness. Third is the supramental transformation in which all becomes supramentalised in the divine gnostic consciousness. It is only with the latter that there can begin the complete transformation of mind, life and body — in my sense of completeness.

The supramental transformation is not the same as the spiritual-mental. It is a change of mind, life and body which the mental or overmental-spiritual cannot achieve. All whom you mention were spirituals, but in different ways. Krishna's mind, for instance, was overmentalised, Ramakrishna's intuitive, Chaitanya's spiritual-psychic, Buddha's illumined higher mental. All that is different from the supramental.

*

The earth-consciousness does not want to change, so it rejects what comes down to it from above — it has always done so. It is only if those who have taken this Yoga open themselves and are willing to change their lower nature that this unwillingness can disappear.

What stands in the way, of course, is always the vital ego with its ignorance and the pride of its ignorance, and the physical consciousness with its inertia which resents and resists any call to change and its indolence which does not like to take the trouble — it finds it more comfortable to go on its own way repeating always the same old movements and, at best, expecting everything to be done for it in some way at some time.

The first thing is to have the right inner attitude — the rest is the will to transform oneself and the vigilance to perceive and reject all that belongs to the ego and the tamasic persistence of the lower nature. Finally, to keep oneself always open to the Mother in every part of the being so that the process of transformation may find no hindrance.

*

This Yoga does not mean a rejection of the powers of life, but an inner transformation and a change of the spirit in the life and the use of the powers. These powers are now used in an egoistic spirit and for undivine ends; they have to be used in a spirit of surrender to the Divine and for the purposes of the divine work. That is what is meant by conquering them back for the Mother.

The life and work developing here in the Ashram has to deal with the world problem and has therefore to meet, it could not avoid, the conflict with the working of the hostile Powers in the human being.

*

The boon that we have asked from the Supreme is the greatest that the earth can ask from the Highest, the change that is most difficult to realise, the most exacting in its conditions. It is nothing less than the descent of the supreme Truth and Power into Matier, the supramental established in the material plane and consciousness and the material world and an integral transformation down to the very principle of Matter. Only a supreme Grace can effect this miracle.

*

A total surrender, an exclusive self-opening to the divine influence, a constant and integral choice of the Truth and rejection of the falsehood, these are the only conditions made. To be one with the Eternal is the object of Yoga; there is no other object. All other aims are included in this one divine perfection.

*

If our seeking is for a total perfection of the being, the physical part of it cannot be left aside; for the body is the material basis, the body is the instrument which we have to use. A total perfection is the ultimate aim which we set before us, for our ideal is the Divine Life which we wish to create here, the life of the Spirit fulfilled on earth, life accomplishing its own spiritual transformation even here on earth in the conditions of the material nature.

We want an integral transformation, the transformation of the body and all its activities. But there is a first step, absolutely indispensable, which has to be completed before anything else can be undertaken; it is the transformation of the consciousness. The starting-point, it goes without saying, is the aspiration towards this transformation and the will to realise it; without that nothing can be done. But if to the aspiration is added an inner opening, a kind of receptivity, then one can enter at a bound into this transformed consciousness and remain there. It is a complete and absolute change, a revolution in the basic poise; it is somewhat like turning a ball inside out. In the changed consciousness everything appears not only new and different, but almost the reverse of what it looked like to the ordinary consciousness. In the transformed consciousness, you start from knowledge, and proceed from knowledge to knowledge. Yet it is only a beginning. Different parts and planes of the being are transformed slowly and gradually as the result of an inner transformation.

*

It is absolutely idle to think of transforming the body when other things that are so much easier to do — though, of course, none is easy — are not done. The inner must change before the outermost can follow. What has to be done with the body at first is to make it open to the Force, so as to receive strength against illness and fatigue — when they come, there must be the power to react and throw them off and to keep a constant flow of force into the body. If that is done, the rest of the bodily change can wait for its proper time.

The Mother:

Governments succeed governments, regimes follow regimes, centuries pass after centuries, but human misery remains lamentably the same. It will always be so, as long as man remains what he is, blind and ignorant, closed to all spiritual reality. A transformation, an illumination of the human consciousness alone can bring about a real amelioration in the condition of humanity. Thus even from the standpoint of human life, it follows logically that the first duty of man is to seek and possess the divine consciousness.

*

In the integral Yoga, the integral life down even to the smallest detail has to be transformed, to be divinised.

VIOLENCE — NON-VIOLENCE

There is a truth in Ahimsa, there is a truth in destruction also. I do not teach that you should go on killing everybody every day as a spiritual dharma. I say that destruction can be done when it is part of the divine work commanded by the Divine. Non-violence is better than violence as a rule, and still sometimes violence may be the right thing. I consider dharma as relative; unity with the Divine and action from the Divine Will, the highest way.

Destruction in itself is neither good nor evil. It is a fact of Nature, a necessity in the play of forces, as things are in this world.

*

But the Gita, which strongly insists on a perfect and absolute samata, goes on to say, "Fight, destroy the adversary, conquer". If there is no kind of general action wanted, no loyalty to Truth as against Falsehood except for one's personal sadhana, no will for the Truth to conquer, then the samata of indifference will suffice. But here there is a work to be done, a Truth to be established against which immense forces are arranged, invisible forces which can use visible things and persons and actions for their instruments. If one is among the disciples, the seeker of this Truth, one has to take sides for the Truth, to stand against the forces that attack it and seek to stifle it. It is personal and egoistic feeling that has to be thrown away, hatred and vital ill-will have to be rejected. It is a principle of action that has to be seen in its right light and proportions.

SECTION THREE

PRAYERS AND MEDITATIONS OF THE MOTHER

Our artificial and exterior way of seeing and understanding is, if it may be so said, foreign to Thee, opposed to Thy nature.

*

All my thoughts go towards Thee, all my acts are consecrated to Thee; Thy Presence is for me an absolute, immutable, invariable fact, and Thy Peace dwells constantly in my heart. Yet I know that this state of union is poor and precarious compared with that which it will become possible for me to realise tomorrow, and I am as yet far, no doubt very far, from that identification in which I shall totally lose the notion of the "I".

*

The daily activity is the anvil on which all the elements must pass and re-pass in order to be purified, refined, made supple and ripe for the illumination which contemplation gives to them. Therefore are pride and satisfaction with oneself the worst of all obstacles.

*

So long as one element of the being, one movement of the thought is still subjected to outside influences, not solely under Thine, it cannot be said that the true Union is realised.

*

In Peace and Silence the Eternal manifests: allow nothing to disturb you and the Eternal will manifest; have perfect equality in face of all and the Eternal will be there. We should not put too much intensity, too much effort into our seeking for Thee; the effort and intensity become a veil in front of Thee: we must not desire to see Thee, for that is still a mental agitation which obscures Thy Eternal Presence; it is in the most complete Peace, Serenity and Equality that all is Thou even as Thou art all. No haste, no inquietude, no tension. And that is better than all the meditations in the world.

*

Like a flame that burns in silence, like a perfume that rises straight upward without wavering, my love goes to Thee; and like the child who does not reason and has no care, I trust myself to Thee that Thy Will may be done.

*

To abide always in Thee is the one thing that matters, always and ever more and more in Thee, beyond illusions and the deceptions of the senses, but living Thee alone in the act whatever it may be; then the illusion is dispelled, the falsehoods of the senses vanish, the bond of consequences is broken, all is transformed into a manifestation of the glory of Thy Eternal Presence.

*

The power of the vital should be mistrusted, it is a tempter on the path of the work, and there is always a risk of falling into its trap, for it gives you the taste of immediate results. Very soon it deflects all our action from the right course and introduces a seed of illusion and death into what we do.

*

To be constantly and integrally at one with Thee is to have the assurance that we shall overcome every obstacle and triumph over all difficulties, both within and without.

*

Even he who might have arrived at perfect contemplation in silence and solitude, could only have done so by extracting himself from his body, by making an abstraction of himself; and thus the substance of which the body is constituted would remain as impure, as imperfect as before, since he would have abandoned it to itself; by a misguided mysticism, by the attraction of supraphysical splendours, by the egoistic desire of being united with Thee for his personal satisfaction, he would have turned his back upon the reason of his earthly existence, he would have refused coward-like to accomplish his mission to redeem and purify Matter. To know that a part of our being is perfectly pure, to commune with that purity, to be identified with it, can be useful only if we subsequently utilise this knowledge for hastening the earthly transfiguration, for accomplishing Thy sublime work.

*

Be more supple, more confident. The only thing thou hast to do is not to let thyself be troubled by anything. To torment oneself about doing good brings about as bad results as bad will. It is in the calm of deep waters that lies the sole possibility of True Service.

*

All is Thine, O Lord, it is Thou who placest everything at our disposal; but how great is our blindness when we imagine that we can be the owners of anything!

*

Those who follow the path of the intellect can have a conception very high and very true; they can conceive the true life, the life one with Thee, but they do not know it; they have no inner experience of that life and they are unaware of any contact with Thee. These, who have an intellectual knowledge and who have shut themselves up for action in a construction which appears to them the best, are the most difficult of all to convert; one finds it harder to awaken in them the consciousness of the Divine than in any other being of good-will.

*

We must at each moment shake off the past like falling dust, so that it may not soil the virgin path which, also at each moment, opens before us.

*

It is in oneself that there are all the obstacles, it is in oneself that there are all the difficulties, it is in oneself that there is all the darkness and ignorance .... The one thing important is to know and obey Thy law with love and joy.

*

We must not run away from suffering, we must not love and cultivate it either, we must learn how to go down deep enough in it to make it a lever which will have the power to force open the doors of the eternal consciousness and enter into the serenity of Thy unvarying oneness.

*

What do the outer circumstances matter ? They appear to me everyday more vain and more illusory, and I take less and less interest in what will outwardly happen to us; but I am more and more intensely interested in the only thing which appears to me important: to know Thee better in order to serve Thee better.

*

O Lord, give us the capacity to do the work without being attached to it, and to develop the powers of individual manifestation without living in the illusion of the personality.

*

Certainly, it is easier to suppress than to organise; but a harmonious order is a realisation far superior to suppression.

*

Terrestrial realisations easily assume a great importance in our eyes, for they are proportioned to our external being, to this limited form which makes of us men. But what is a terrestrial realisation compared with Thee, in front of Thee? However perfect, however complete, however divine it may be, it is only an indiscernible moment in Thy eternity; and the results obtained by it, however powerful, however marvellous they may be, are but an imperceptible atom in the infinite advance towards Thee. It is this that Thy workers should never forget, otherwise they will become unfit to serve Thee.

*

O Divine Master, let Thy light fall upon this chaos and a new world emerge from it. What is now preparing accomplish and let a new humanity be born which will be the perfect expression of Thy new sublime Law.

*

Lord, may Thy will be done, may Thy work be accomplished.

Fortify our devotion, increase our surrender and enlighten us on the path. We establish Thee as the supreme Master within us so that Thou mayst become the Supreme Master of the whole earth.

*

O Lord, if my understanding is limited, widen it; if my knowledge is obscure, enlighten it; if my heart is empty of ardour, set it aflame; if my love is insignificant, make it intense; if my feelings are ignorant and egoistic, give them the full consciousness in the Truth.

*

At every moment we must know how to lose everything in order to gain everything, to shed the past as a dead body and be reborn into a greater plenitude.

*

But when I turn my look towards the earth, I see that man's field of action, however large it may be, is always terribly restricted. A man, who, in his mind and even in his vital being is vast like the universe, or at least like the earth, as soon as he begins to act, is shut up within the narrow limits of a material action, very bounded in its field and results.

*

There is a Power which no government can command, a Happiness which no earthly success can give, a Light which no wisdom can possess, a Knowledge which no philosophy, no science can acquire, a Beatitude of which no satisfaction of desire can give the enjoyment, a thirst for Love which no human relation can quench, a Peace which can be found nowhere, not even in death.

It is the Power, the Happiness, the Light, the Knowledge, the

Beatitude, the Love and the Peace which come to us from the Divine Grace.

*

The heavens have been definitively conquered, and nothing and nobody has the power to take them from me. But the conquest of the earth has yet to be made ....

31-7-1915

*

O my Lord, my sweet Master, for the accomplishment of Thy work I have sunk down into the unfathomble depths of Matter, I have touched with my finger the horror of the falsehood and the inconscience, I have reached the seat of oblivion and a supreme obscurity! But in my heart was the Remembrance, from my heart there leaped the call which could arrive to Thee: "Lord, Lord, everywhere Thy enemies are triumphant; falsehood is the monarch of the world; life without Thee is death, a perpetual hell; doubt has usurped the place of Hope and revolt has pushed out submission; Faith is spent, Gratitude is not born; blind passions and murderous instincts and a guilty weakness have covered and stifled Thy sweet law of love. Lord, wilt Thou permit Thy enemies to prevail, falsehood and ugliness and suffering to triumph? Lord, give the command to conquer and victory will be there. I know we are unworthy, I know the world is not yet ready. But I cry to Thee with an absolute faith in Thy Grace and I know that Thy Grace will save us."

Thus, my prayer rushed up towards Thee: and, from the depths of the abyss, I beheld Thee in Thy radiant splendour; Thou didst appear and Thou saidst to me: "Lose not courage, be firm, be confident, — I COME."

24-11-1931

THE SYNTHESIS OF YOGA

He who chooses the Infinite has been chosen by the Infinite....

For the Sadhaka of the integral Yoga it is necessary to remember that no written Shastra, however great its authority or however large its spirit, can be more that a partial expression of the eternal knowledge. He will use, but never bind himself even by the greatest Scripture. An integral and synthetic Yoga needs especially not to be bound by any written or traditional Shastra; for while it embraces the knowledge received from the past, it seeks to organise it anew for the present and the future....

By this Yoga we not only seek the Infinite, but we call upon the Infinite to unfold himself in human life....

The development of the experience in its rapidity, its amplitude, the intensity and power of its results, depends primarily, in the beginning of the path and long after, on the aspiration and personal effort of the sadhaka. The first determining element of the siddhi is, therefore, the intensity of the turning, the force which directs the soul inward. The power of aspiration of the heart, the force of the will, the concentration of the mind, the perseverance and determination of the applied energy are the measure of that intensity....

So long as the contact with the Divine is not in some considerable degree established, so long as there is not some measure of sustained identity, the element of the personal effort must normally predominate....

Man demands miracles that he may have faith; he wishes to be dazzled in order that he may see. And this impatience, this ignorance may turn into a great danger and disaster if, in our revolt against the divine leading, we call in another distorting Force more satisfying to our impulses and desires and ask it to guide us and give it the Divine Name.

The spiritual progress of most human beings demands an extraneous support, an object of faith outside us. It needs an external image of God; or it needs a human representative, — Incarnation, Prophet or Guru; or it demands both and receives them.

For according to the need of the human soul the Divine manifests himself as deity, as human divine or in simple humanity — using that thick disguise, which so successfully conceals the Godhead, for a means of transmission of his guidance....

All Yoga is in its nature a new birth; it is a birth out of the ordinary, the mentalised material life of man into a higher spiritual consciousness and a greater and diviner being. No Yoga can be successfully undertaken and followed unless there is a strong awakening to the necessity of that larger spiritual existence....

The mere idea or intellectual seeking of something higher beyond, however strongly grasped by the mind's interest, is ineffective unless it is seized on by the heart as the one thing desirable and by the will as the one thing to be done. For truth of the Spirit has not to be merely thought but to be lived, and to live it demands a unified single-mindedness of the being; so great a change as is contemplated by the Yoga is not to be effected by a divided will or by a small portion of the energy or by a hesitating mind. He who seeks the Divine must consecrate himself to God and to God only....

But for the sadhaka of the integral Yoga, in accepting life, he has to bear not only his own burden, but a great part of the world's burden too along with it, as a continuation of his own sufficiently heavy load. Therefore his Yoga has much more of the nature of a battle than other's; but this is not only an individual battle, it is a collective war waged over a considerable country. He has not only to conquer in himself the forces of egoistic falsehood and disorder, but to conquer them as a representative of the same adverse and inexhaustible forces in the world....

The transformation of our superficial, narrow and fragmentary human way of thinking, seeing, feeling and being into a deep and wide spiritual consciousness and an integrated inner and outer existence and of our ordinary human living into the divine way of life must be its central purpose. The means towards this supreme end is a self-giving of all our nature to the Divine ....

The life of the human creature, as it is ordinarily lived, is composed of a half-fixed, half-fluid mass of very imperfectly ruled thoughts, perceptions, sensations, emotions, desires, enjoyments, acts mostly customary and self-repeating, in part only dynamic and self-developing, but all centred around a superficial ego. The sum of movement of these activities eventuates in an internal growth which is partly visible and operative in this life, partly a seed of progress in lives hereafter. This growth of the conscious being, an expansion, an increasing self-expression, a more and more harmonised development of his constituent members is the whole meaning and all the pith of human existence. It is for this meaningful development of consciousness by thought, will, emotion, desire, action and experience, leading in the end to a supreme divine self-discovery, that Man, the mental being, has entered into the material body. The aim set before our Yoga is nothing less than to hasten this supreme object of our existence here. It is this new birth that we make our aim: a growth into a divine consciousness is the whole meaning of our Yoga, an integral conversion to divinity not only of the soul but of all the parts of our nature....

The Gita at its cryptic close may seem by its silence to stop short of that solution for which we are seeking; it pauses at the borders of the highest spiritual mind and does not cross them into the splendours of the supramental Light....

The true essence of sacrifice is not self-immolation, it is self-giving; its object not self-effacement, but self-fulfilment; its method not self-mortification, but a greater life, not self-mutilation, but a transformation of our natural human parts into divine members, not self-torture, but a passage from a lesser satisfaction to a greater Ananda....

To the soul that wholly gives itself to him, God also gives himself altogether. Only the one who offers his whole nature, finds the Self. Only the one who can give everything, enjoys the Divine All everywhere. Only a supreme self-abandonment attains to the Supreme. Only the sublimation by sacrifice of all that we are, can enable us to embody the Highest and live here in the immanent consciousness of the transcendent Spirit....

The practice of this Yoga of sacrifice compels us to renounce all the inner supports of egoism, casting them out of our mind and will and actions, and to eliminate its seed, its presence, its influence out of our nature. All must be done for the Divine; all must be directed towards the Divine. Nothing must be attempted for ourselves as a separate existence; nothing done for others, whether neighbours, friends, family, country or mankind or other creatures merely because they are connected with our personal life and thought and sentiment or because the ego takes a preferential interest in their welfare....

This pilgrimage of ascension and this descent for the labour of transformation must be inevitably a battle, a long war with ourselves and with opposing forces around us which, while it lasts, may well seem interminable. For all our old obscure and ignorant nature will contend repeatedly and obstinately with the transforming Influence, supported in its lagging unwillingness or its stark resistance by most of the established forces of environing universal Nature; the powers and principalities and the ruling beings of the Ignorance will not easily give up their empire....

It is for this that a surrender and submission to That which is beyond us enabling the full and free working of its Power is indispensable. As that self-giving progresses, the work of the sacrifice becomes easier and more powerful and the prevention of the opposing Forces loses much of its strength, impulsion and substance....

The extreme solution insisted on by the world-shunning ascetic or the inward-turned ecstatical and self-oblivious mystic is evidently foreign to the purpose of an integral Yoga; for if we are to realise the Divine in the world, it cannot be done by leaving aside the world-action and action itself altogether. The spiritualisation of both the inward being and the outward life and not a compromise between life and the spirit is the goal of which we are the seekers....

The guiding law of spiritual experience can only come by an opening of human consciousness to the Divine Consciousness; there must be the power to receive in us the working and command and dynamic presence of the Divine Shakti and surrender ourselves to her control; it is that surrender and that control which bring the guidance....

The integral Yoga, refusing to rely upon the fragile stuff of mental and moral ideals, puts its whole emphasis in this field on three central dynamic processes — the development of the true soul or psychic being to take the place of the false soul of desire, the sublimation of human into divine love, the elevation of consciousness from its mental to its spiritual and supramental plane by whose power alone both the soul and the life-force can be utterly delivered from the veils and prevarications of the Ignorance....

This physical mind of inertia of the ignorant man believes in no divinity other than its small earth-gods; it aspires perhaps to a greater comfort, order, pleasure, but asks for no uplifting and spiritual deliverance. A principle of dark and dull inertia is at its base; all are tied down by the body and its needs and desires to a trivial mind, petty desires and emotions, an insignificant repetition of small worthless functionings, needs, cares, occupations, pains, pleasures that lead to nothing beyond themselves and bear the stamp of an ignorance that knows not its own why and whither....

Life is indispensable to the completeness of the creative spiritual realisation, but life released, transformed, uplifted, not the ordinary mentalised human-animal life, nor the demoniac or Titanic, not even the divine and the undivine mixed together. If once our consciousness could reach the heights of a supramental Nature, then indeed these disabilities would disappear....

The integral Yoga cannot reject the works of Life and be satisfied with an inward experience only; it has to go inward in order to change the outward, making the Life-Force a part and a working of a Yoga-Energy which is in touch with the Divine and divine in its guidance....

The soul of desire is a separative soul of ego and all its instincts are for a separative self-affirmation. It is when there is this death of desire and this calm equal wideness in the consciousness everywhere, that the true vital being within us comes out from the veil and reveals its own calm, intense and potent presence....

A call of the veiled psychic element oppressed by the mass of the outer ignorance and crying for deliverance, a stress of eager meditation and seeking for knowledge, a longing of the heart, a passionate will ignorant yet but sincere may break the lid that shuts off the Higher from the Lower Nature and open the flood-gates....

Whoever clings to the desires and weaknesses of the flesh, the cravings and passions of the vital in its turbulent ignorance, the dictates of his personal mind unsilenced and unillumined by a greater knowledge, cannot find the true inner law and is heaping obstacles in the way of the divine fulfilment. Whoever is able to detect and renounce those obscuring agencies and to discern and follow the true Guide within and without will discover the spiritual law and reach the goal of the Yoga....

The good is all that helps the individual and the world towards their divine fullness, and evil is all that retards or breaks up that increasing perfection....

To those who can act only on a rigid standard, to those who can feel only the human and not the divine values, this truth may seem to be a dangerous concession which is likely to destroy the very foundation of morality, confuse all conduct and establish only chaos....

The true business of man upon earth is to express in the type of humanity a growing image of the Divine; whether knowingly or unknowingly, it is to this end that Nature is working in him under the thick veil of her inner and outer processes. But the material or animal man is ignorant of the inner aim of life; he knows only its needs and its desires and he has necessarily no other guide to what is required of him than his own perception of need and his own stirrings and pointings of desire....

Whoever sincerely enters the path of works, must leave behind him the stage in which need and desire are the first law of our acts. For whatever desires still trouble his being, he must, if he accepts the high aim of Yoga, put them away from him into the hands of the Lord within us. The supreme Power will deal with them for the good of the sadhaka and for the good of all....

The total surrender, then, of all our actions to a supreme and universal Will, an unconditioned and standardless surrender of all works to the government of something eternal within us which will replace the ordinary working of the ego-nature, is the way and end of Karmayoga....

An entire self-consecration, a complete equality, an unsparing effacement of the ego, a transforming deliverance of the nature from its ignorant modes of action are the steps by which the surrender of all the being and nature to the Divine Will can be prepared and achieved, — a self-giving true, total and without reserve....

So long as we work with attachment to the result, the sacrifice is offered not to the Divine, but to our ego. We may think otherwise, but we are deceiving ourselves; we are making our idea of the Divine, our sense of duty, our feeling for our fellow-creatures, our idea of what is good for the world or others, even our obedience to the Master a mask for our egoistic satisfactions and preferences and a spacious shield against the demand made on us to root all desire out of our natures....

At this stage of the Yoga and even throughout the Yoga this form of desire, this figure of the ego is the enemy against whom we have to be always on our guard with an unsleeping vigilance....

It is still the "I" that chooses and determines, it is still the "I" that undertakes the responsibility and feels the demerit or the merit. An entire removal of this separative ego-sense is an essential aim of our Yoga.

The sadhaka has not only to think and know but to see and feel concretely and intensely even in the moment of the working and in its initiation and whole process that his works are not his at all, but are coming through him from the Supreme Existence. He must be always aware of a Force, a Presence, a Will that acts through his individual nature....

A great sincerity is asked for and has to be imposed not only on the conscious mind but still more on the subliminal part of us which is full of hidden movements. For there is there, especially in our subliminal vital nature, an incorrigible charlatan and actor. The sadhaka must first have advanced far in the elimination of desire and in the firm equality of his soul towards all workings and all happenings before he can utterly lay down the burden of his works on the Divine. At every moment he must proceed with a vigilant eye upon the deceits of the ego and the ambushes of the misleading Powers of Darkness. Wherever desire and ego harbour, passion and disturbance harbour with them and share their life....

The Master of the work does not reveal himself at once to the seeker. Always it is his Power that acts behind the veil, but it is manifest only when we renounce the egoism of the worker, and its direct movement increases in proportion as that renunciation becomes more and more concrete. Only when our surrender to his divine Shakti is absolute, shall we have the right to live in his absolute presence....

There must, therefore, be stages and gradations in our approach to this perfection, as there are in the progress towards all other perfection on any plane of Nature....

In all Yogas the first requisites are faith and patience. And in the long and difficult integral Yoga there must be an integral faith and an unshakable patience....

The Master of our works respects our nature even when he is transforming it; he works always through the nature and not by any arbitrary caprice....

The rules which the intellect of men lays down cannot apply to the liberated soul, — by the external criteria and tests which their mental association and prejudgments prescribe, such a one cannot be judged; he is outside the narrow jurisdiction of these fallible tribunals. He is not governed by the judgments of men or the laws laid down by the ignorant; he obeys an inner voice and is moved by an unseen Power....

To participate in the divine work, to live for God in the world will be the rule of the Karmayogin; to live for God in the world and therefore so to act that the Divine may more and more manifest himself and the world go forward by whatever way of its obscure pilgrimage and move nearer to the divine ideal....

*

A free heart is a heart delivered from the gusts and storms of the affections and the passions; the assailing touch of grief, wrath, hatred, fear, inequality of love, trouble of joy, pain of sorrow fall away from the equal heart, and leave it a thing large, calm, equal, luminous, divine....

*

To be self-ruler is not possible for him if he is subject to the attacks of the lower nature, to the turbulence of grief and joy, to the violent touches of pleasure and pain, to the tumult of his emotions and passions, to the bondage of his personal likings and dislikings, to the strong chains of desire and attachment, to the narrowness of a personal and emotionally preferential judgment and opinion, to all the hundred touches of his egoism and its pursuing stamp on his thought, feeling and action. All these things are the slavery to the lower self which the greater "I" in man must put under his feet if he is to be king of his own nature. To surmount them is the condition of self-rule, but of that surmounting again equality is the condition and the essence of the movement.

THE DIVINE LIFE

Our endeavour has been to discover what is the reality and significance of our existence as conscious beings in the material universe and in what direction and how far that significance once discovered leads us, to what human or divine future....

But consciousness as it is, life as it is cannot be the whole secret; for both are very clearly something unfinished and still in process.

In us consciousness is Mind and our mind is ignorant and imperfect, an intermediate power that has grown and is still growing towards something beyond itself.... Before our thinking, reasoning, reflecting mind there was a consciousness unthinking but living and sentient, and before that there was the sub-conscious and the unconscious; after us or in our yet unevolved selves there is likely to be waiting a greater consciousness, self-luminous, not dependent on constructive thought: our imperfect and ignorant thought-mind is certainly not the last word of consciousness, its ultimate possibility.... Its destiny must be to evolve into its own perfection which is its true nature.... The destiny of evolving consciousness must be, then, to become perfect in its awareness, entirely aware of self and all-aware.... It is this to which we have given the name of Supermind or Gnosis....

If consciousness is the central secret, life is the outward indication, the effective power of being in Matter; for it is that which liberates consciousness and gives it its form or embodiment of force and its effectuation in material act.... Man, the mental being, has an imperfect life because mind is not the first and highest power of consciousness of the Being; even if mind were perfected, there would be still something yet to be realised, not yet manifested. For what is involved and emergent is not a Mind, but a Spirit, and mind is not the native dynamism of consciousness of the Spirit; supermind, the light of gnosis, is its native dynamism. If then life has to become a manifestation of the Spirit, it is the manifestation of a spiritual being in us and the divine life of a perfected consciousness in a supramental or gnostic power of spiritual being that must be the secret burden and intention of evolutionary Nature....

As the mind and life become illumined with the light of the spirit, they put on or reflect something of the divinity, the secret greater Reality.... But, for the full and perfect fulfilment of the evolutionary urge, this illumination and change must take up and re-create the whole being, mind, life and body ... it must take form not only in the life of the individual but as a collective life or gnostic beings established as a highest power and form of the becoming of the Spirit in the earth-nature.... There can undoubtedly be a spiritual life within, a kingdom of heaven within us which is not dependent on any outer manifestation or instrumentation or formula of external being. The inner life has a supreme spiritual importance and the outer has a value only in so far as it is expressive of the inner status....

In our present life of Nature, in our externalised surface existence, it is the world that seems to create us; but in the turn to the spiritual life it is we who must create ourselves and our world. In this new formula of creation, the inner life becomes of the first importance and the rest can be only its expression and outcome....

In the growth into a divine life the spirit must be our first preoccupation; until we have revealed and evolved it in our self out of its mental, vital, physical wrappings and disguises, extricated it with patience from our own body, as the Upanishad puts it, until we have built up in ourselves an inner life of the spirit, it is obvious that no outer divine living can become possible.... A perfected human world cannot be created by men or composed of men who are themselves imperfect....

This then is the first necessity that the individual, each individual, shall discover the spirit, the divine reality within him and express that in all his being and living. A divine life must be first and foremost an inner life; for since the outward must be the expression of what is within, there can be no divinity in the outer existence if there is not the divinisation of the inner being.... To be aware wholly and integrally of oneself and of all the truth of one's being is the necessary condition of true possession of existence. This self-awareness is what is meant by spiritual knowledge....

To become complete in being, in consciousness of being, in force of being, in delight of being and to live in this integrated completeness is the divine living.... All being is one and to be fully is to be all that is. To be in the being of all and to include all in one's being, to be conscious of the consciousness of all, to be integrated in force with the universal force, to carry all action and experience, in oneself and feel it as one's own action and experience, to feel all selves as one's own self, to feel all delight of being as one's own delight of being is a necessary condition of the integral divine living....

But thus to be universally in the fullness and freedom of one's universality, one must be also transcendentally. The spiritual fullness of the being is eternity; if one has not the consciousness of timeless eternal being, if one is dependent on body or embodied mind or embodied life, or dependent on this world or that world or on this condition of being or that condition of being, that is not the reality of self, not the fullness of our spiritual existence. To live only as a self of body or be only by the body is to be an ephemeral creature, subject to death and desire and pain and suffering and decay and decadence. To transcend, to exceed consciousness of body, not to be held in the body or by the body, to hold the body only as an instrument, a minor outward formation of self, is a first condition of divine living....

He must enter into the supreme divine Reality, feel his oneness with it, live in it, be its self-creation: all his mind, life, physicality must be converted into terms of its Supernature.

These things are impossible without an inward living; they cannot be reached by remaining in an external consciousness turned always outwards, active only or mainly on and from the surface. The individual being has to find himself, his true existence; he can only do this by going inward, by living within and from within: for the external or outer consciousness or life separated from the inner spirit is the field of the Ignorance....

This movement of going inward and living inward is a difficult task to lay upon the normal consciousness of the human being; yet there is no other way of self-finding....

But to those into whose composition there has entered the power of a more inner living, the movement of going within and living within brings not a darkness or dull emptiness but an enlargement, a rush of new experience, a greater vision, a larger capacity, an extended life infinitely more real and various than the first pettiness of the life constructed for itself by our normal physical humanity, a joy of being which is larger and richer than any delight in existence that the outer vital man or the surface mental man can gain by their dynamic vital force and activity or subtlety and expansion of the mental existence. A silence, an entry into a wide or even immense or infinite emptiness is part of the inner spiritual experience...it is the passage not into non-existence but to a greater existence.

Our utmost universalisation on the surface is a poor and limping endeavour, — it is a construction, a make-believe and not the real thing; for in our surface consciousness we are bound to separation of consciousness from others and wear the fetters of the ego. There our very selflessness becomes more often than not a subtle form of selfishness or turns into a larger affirmation of our ego; content with our pose of altruism, we do not see that it is a veil for the imposition of our individual self, our ideas, our mental and vital personality, our need of ego-enlargement upon the others whom we take up into our expanded orbit....

.... The gnostic being will act, not out of a surface sentiment of love and sympathy or any similar feeling, but out of this close mutual consciousness, this intimate oneness. All his action in the world will be enlightened by a truth of vision of what has to be done, a sense of the will of the Divine Reality in him which is also the Divine Reality in others, and it will be done for the Divine in all for the effectuation of the truth of purpose of the All as seen in the light of the highest Consciousness and in the way and by the steps through which it must be effectuated in the power of the Supernature.... There is no separative ego in him to initiate anything; it is the Transcendent and Universal that moves out through his universalised individuality into the action of the universe. As he does not live for a separate ego, so too he does not live for the purpose of any collective ego; he lives in and for the Divine in himself, in and for the Divine in the collectivity, in and for the Divine in all beings. This universality in action, organised by the all-seeing Will in the sense of the realised oneness of all, is the law of his divine living.... This calls for the appearance not only of isolated evolved individuals acting in the unevolved mass, but of many gnostic individuals forming a new kind of beings and a new common life superior to the present individual and common existence....

All will be united by the evolution of the Truth-consciousness in them; in the changed way of being which this consciousness would bring about in them, they will feel themselves to be embodiments of a single self, souls of a single Reality....

Unity is the basis of the gnostic consciousness, mutuality the natural result of its direct awareness of oneness in diversity, harmony the inevitable power of the working of its force. Unity, mutuality and harmony must therefore be the inescapable law of a common or collective gnostic life....

An evolution of innate and latent but as yet unevolved powers of consciousness is not considered admissible by the modern mind, because these exceed our present formulation of Nature and, to our ignorant preconceptions founded on a limited experience, they seem to belong to the supernatural, to the miraculous and occult; for they surpass the known action of material Energy which is now ordinarily accepted as the sole cause and mode of things and the sole instrumentation of the World-Force.... But there would be nothing supernatural or miraculous in such an evolution, except in so far as it would be a supernature or superior nature to ours just as human nature is a supernature or superior nature to that of animal or plant or material objects....

What is lacking is a spiritual knowledge and spiritual power, a power over self, a power born of inner unification with others, a power over the surrounding or invading world-forces, a full-visioned and fully equipped power of effectuation of knowledge; it is these capacities missing or defective in us that belong to the very substance of gnostic being, for they are inherent in the light and dynamis of the gnostic nature....

Our nature is complex and we have to find a key to some perfect unity and fullness of its complexity. Its first evolutionary basis is the material life; Nature began with that and man also has to begin with it; he has first to affirm his material and vital existence. But if he stops there, there can be for him no evolution; his next and greater preoccupation must be to find himself as a mental being in a material life — both individual and social — as perfected as possible.... Beyond and above this preoccupation, as soon as mind is sufficiently developed, there awakes in man the spiritual preoccupation, the discovery of a self and inmost truth of being and the release of man's mind and life into the truth of the Spirit, its perfection by the power of the Spirit, the solidarity, unity, mutuality of all beings in the Spirit....

As an element in the total complexity of human life, this stress on a perfected economic and material existence has its place in the whole: as a sole or predominant stress it is for humanity itself, for the evolution itself full of danger. The first danger is a resurgence of the old vital and material primitive barbarian in a civilised form; the means Science has put at our disposal eliminates the peril of the subversion and destruction of an effete civilisation by stronger primitive peoples, but it is the resurgence of the barbarian in ourselves, in civilised man, that is the peril, and this we see all around us. For that is bound to come if there is no high and strenuous mental and moral ideal controlling and uplifting the vital and physical man in us and no spiritual ideal liberating him from himself into his inner being....

At present mankind is undergoing an evolutionary crisis in which is concealed a choice of its destiny; for a stage has been reached in which the human mind has achieved in certain directions an enormous development while in others it stands arrested and bewildered and can no longer find its way.... Man has created a system of civilisation which has become too big for his limited mental capacity and understanding and his still more limited spiritual and moral capacity to utilise and manage, a too dangerous servant of his blundering ego and its appetites....

A life of unity, mutuality and harmony born of a deeper and wider truth of our being is the only truth of life that can successfully replace the imperfect mental constructions of the past which were a combination of association and regulated conflict, an accommodation of egos and interests grouped or dovetailed into each other to form a society, a consolidation by common general life-motives, a unification by need and the pressure of struggle with outside forces....

A total spiritual direction given to the whole life and the whole nature can alone lift humanity beyond itself.... It is only the full emergence of the soul, the full descent of the native light and power of the Spirit and consequent replacement or transformation and uplifting of our insufficient mental and vital nature by a spiritual and supramental supernature that can effect this evolutionary miracle ... what evolutionary Nature presses for, is an awakening to the knowledge of self, the discovery of self, the manifestation of the self and spirit within us and the release of its self-knowledge, its self-power, its native self-instrumentation....

What is necessary is that there should be a turn in humanity felt by some or many towards the vision of this change, a feeling of its imperative need, the sense of its possibility, the will to make it possible in themselves and to find the way.... The inner change can begin to take shape in a collective form only if the gnostic individual finds others who have the same kind of inner life as himself and can form with them a group with its own autonomous existence or else a separate community or order of beings with its own inner law of life. It is this need of a separate life with its rule of living adapted to the inner power or motive force of the spiritual existence and creating for it its native atmosphere that has expressed itself in the past in the formation of the monastic life or in attempts of various kinds at a new separate collective living self-governed and other in its spiritual principle than the ordinary human life. The monastic life is in its nature an association of other-worldly seekers, men whose whole attempt is to find and realise in themselves the spiritual reality and who form their common existence by rules of living which help them in that endeavour. It is not usually an effort to create a new life-formation which all exceed the ordinary human society and create a new world-order. A religion may hold that eventual prospect before it or attempt some first approach to it, or a mental idealism may make the same endeavour. But these attempts have always been overcome by the persistent inconscience and ignorance of our human vital nature.... Either the endeavour fails by its own imperfection or it is invaded by the imperfection of the outside world and sinks from the shining height of its aspiration to something mixed and inferior on the ordinary human level. A common spiritual life meant to express the spiritual and not the mental, vital and physical being must found and maintain itself on greater values than the mental, vital, physical values of the ordinary human society.... An entirely new consciousness in many individuals transforming their whole being, transforming their mental, vital and physical nature-self, is needed for the new life to appear; only such a transformation of the general mind, life, body nature can bring into being a new worthwhile collective existence....

A general change from the old consciousness taking up the whole life into the spiritual principle would be the necessary first step; the preparation for this might be long and the transformation itself once begun proceed by stages.... At a certain stage it might be necessary to follow the agelong device of the separate community, but with a double purpose, first to provide a secure atmosphere, a place and life apart, in which the consciousness of the individual might concentrate on its evolution in surroundings where all was turned and centred towards the one endeavour and, next, when things were ready, to formulate and develop the new life in those surroundings and this prepared spiritual atmosphere. It might be that, in such a concentration of effort, all the difficulties of the change would present themselves with a concentrated force; for each seeker, carrying in himself the possibilities but also the imperfections of a world that has to be transformed, would bring in not only his capacities but his difficulties and the oppositions of the old nature and, mixed together in the restricted circle of a small and close common life, these might assume a considerably enhanced force of obstruction which would tend to counterbalance the enhanced power and concentration of the forces making for the evolution. This is a difficulty that has broken in the past all the efforts of mental man to evolve something better and more true and harmonious than the ordinary mental and vital life. But if Nature is ready and has taken her evolutionary decision or if the power of the Spirit descending from the higher planes is sufficiently strong, the difficulty would be overcome and a first evolutionary formation or formations would be possible....

A complete seclusion or separation of the life of a spiritual community from the life of the Ignorance would then seem to impose itself: for otherwise a compromise between the two lives would be necessary and with the compromise a danger of contamination or incompleteness of the greater exisence; two different and incompatible principles of existence would be in contact and, even though the greater would influence the lesser, the smaller life would also have its effect on the greater, since such mutual impact is the law of all contiguity and interchange.... But it is to be supposed that the new and completer light would bring also a new and completer power. It might not be necessary for it to be entirely separate; it might establish itself in so many islets and from there spread through the old life, throwing out upon it its own influences and filtrations, gaining upon it, bringing to it a help and illumination which a new aspiration in mankind might after a time begin to understand and welcome....

If we suppose the gnostic consciousness to be established in the earth-life, the power and knowledge at its disposal would be much greater than the power and knowledge of the mental man, and the life of a community of gnostic beings, supposing it to be separate, would be as safe against attack as the organised life of man against any attack by a lower species.... The influence of the supramental principle on earth would fall upon the life of the Ignorance and impose harmony on it within its limits. It is conceivable that the gnostic life would be separate, but it would surely admit within its borders as much of human life as was turned towards spirituality and in progress towards the heights....

As the universalised spiritual individual sheds the limited personality, the ego, as he rises beyond mind to a completer knowledge in Supernature, the conflicting ideals of the mind must fall away from him, but what is true behind them will remain in the life of Supernature. The gnostic consciousness is a consciousness in which all contradictions are cancelled or fused into each other in a higher light of seeing and being, in a unified self-knowledge and world-knowledge. The gnostic being will not accept the mind's ideals and standards; he will not be moved to live for himself, for his ego, or for humanity or for others or for the community or for the State; for he will be aware of something greater than these half-truths, of the Divine Reality, and it is for that he will live....

Life and the body would be no longer tyrannous masters demanding nine-tenths of existence for their satisfaction, but means and powers for the expression of the spirit. At the same time, since the matter and the body are accepted, the control and the right use of physical things would be a part of the realised life of the spirit in the manifestation in earth-nature.... A complete purity and self-mastery would be in the very grain of its nature and that would remain the same in poverty or in riches.... The one rule of the gnostic life would be the self-expression of the Spirit, the will of the Divine Being....

A life of gnostic beings carrying the evolution to a higher supramental status might fitly be characterised as a divine life; for it would be a life in the Divine....

It must lead inevitably towards an evolution in the Knowledge, a self-finding and self-unfolding of the Spirit, a self-revelation of the Divinity in things in that true power of itself in Nature which is to us still a Supernature.

APPENDIX

THE PASSING OF SRI AUROBINDO AND HIS RETURN

The Mother:

To THEE who hast been the material envelope of our Master, to THEE our infinite gratitude. Before THEE who hast done so much for us, who hast worked, struggled, suffered, hoped, endured so much, before THEE who hast willed all, attempted all, prepared, achieved all for us, before THEE we bow down and implore that we may never forget, even for a moment, all we owe to THEE.

9-12-1950

*

The lack of receptivity of the earth and men is mostly responsible for the decision Sri Aurobindo has taken regarding his body. But one thing is certain; what has happened on the physical plane affects in no way the truth of his teaching. All that he has said is perfectly true and remains so. Time and the course of events will prove it abundantly.

8-12-1950

*

Our Lord has sacrificed himself totally for us.... He was not compelled to leave his body, he chose to do so for reasons so sublime that they are beyond the reach of human mentality. And when one cannot understand, the only thing to do is to keep a respectful silence.

26-12-1950

*

We stand in the Presence of Him who has sacrificed his physical life in order to help more fully his work of transformation.

He is always with us, aware of what we are doing, of all our thoughts, of all our feelings and all our actions.

18-1-1951

*

To grieve is an insult to Sri Aurobindo who is here with us, conscious and alive.

14-12-1950

*

Sri Aurobindo has given up his body in an act of supreme unselfishness, renouncing the realisation in his body to hasten the hour of the collective realisation. Surely if the earth were more responsive, this would not have been necessary.

12-6-1953

*

When I asked him to resuscitate he clearly answered: "I have left this body purposely. I will not take it back. I shall manifest again in the first supramental body built in the supramental way".

8-12-1950

FROM AN ARTICLE, "A CALL FROM PONDICHERRY" BY DR. SANYAL

The Mother came with us into the ante-room and then for the first time declared: "He is fully conscious within but is losing interest in Himself". Dr. Satya Sen was restless as energetic treatment could not be instituted. She simply said: "It all depends on Him".

*

The Mother whispered, "As long as the supramental Light does not pass away, the body will not show any signs of decomposition and it may be a day or it may take more days." I whispered to her, where is the light you speak of — can I not see it? She smiled at me and with infinite compassion put her hand on my head. There he was — with a luminous mantle of bluish golden hue around Him.

*

The Mother said to me, People do not know what a tremendous sacrifice He has made for the world. About a year ago, while I was discussing things, I remarked that I felt like leaving this body of mine. He spoke out in a very firm tone, "No, this can never be. If necessary for this transformation I might go, you will have to fulfil our Yoga of supramental descent and transformation."

*

In my own foolish way I voiced my apprehension for Her health and the strain she put on her fragile frame. She smiled at me and asked, "Do you think I get all this energy from my frugal meals? Of course not, one can draw infinite energy from the universe when needed". She also added, "No, I have no intention of leaving my body for the present. I have yet a lot of things to do. So far as I am concerned, it is nothing to me. I am in constant contact with Sri Aurobindo."

*

I naively asked the Mother, why I was not allowed to treat the

Lord as I would have done in the routine way, and why I was called in? The Mother consoled me by saying, "We wanted you to be here, not so much for treatment".

EXTRACT FROM A RECORD OF TALKS WITH SRI AUROBINDO ON 25-9-1924

We must conserve the energy and use it in rising up to higher life. I have faith in the truth of transformation of life. I have complete faith that it will be achieved. The truth of sexual life can be seen after the complete transformation of the body also. I for one have put the sexual side completely aside so that I may make this daring attempt .... I may not be able to do it completely and a part may be left. But I shall be born again to complete it. The way of reproduction may not be the same as in ordinary life.

FROM AN ARTICLE BY SRI AUROBINDO — 'DIVINE BODY' IN THE YEAR 1949

But yet there may be circumstances in which from another standpoint, a voluntary creation of bodies for souls that seek to enter the earth-life to help in the creation and extension of the divine life on earth might be found to be desirable. Then the necessity of a physical procreation for this purpose could only be avoided if new means of a supra-physical kind were evolved and made available ....

*

It should be possible and it is believed to be possible for an object formed in this subtle physical to make a transit from its subtlety into the state of gross Matter directly by the intervention of an occult force and process whether with or even without the assistance or intervention of some gross material procedure. A soul wishing to enter into a body or form for itself a body and take part in a divine life upon earth might be assisted to do so or even provided with such a form by this method of direct transmutation without passing through birth by the sex-process or undergoing any degradation.

The Mother:

But such as we are, we have been created in the ordinary animal way and therefore even if we are transformed, something of the animal origin will remain. The supramental being, as conceived by Sri Aurobindo, is not at all formed in the ordinary animal way, but directly, by a process which for the moment still appears occult to us; it is a direct handling of the substance and forces in such a way that the body is a materialisation and not a formation following the ordinary animal principle...perhaps it will not be necessary for many years to pass before the first visible results will become apparent to all....

Extracts taken from the following books particularly and from other works of the Master and the Mother:

1. The Mother
2. Lights on Yoga
3. More Lights on Yoga
4. Bases of Yoga
5. The Yoga and Its Objects
6. The Riddle of this World
7. Elements of Yoga
8. Sri Aurobindo on Himself and on The Mother
9. Letters of Sri Aurobindo
10. The Synthesis of Yoga
11. Words of the Mother
12. On Education
13. Prayers and Meditations of the Mother